Measuring

Medical Education

The Tests and the Experience of the
National Board of Medical Examiners

Measuring
Medical Education

The Tests and the Experience of the
National Board of Medical Examiners

SECOND EDITION

JOHN P. HUBBARD, M.D.

President Emeritus, National Board of Medical Examiners
Professor Emeritus, University of Pennsylvania School of Medicine

with chapters by members of the staff,
National Board of Medical Examiners

BARBARA J. ANDREW, Ph.D.

Director, Department of Research and Development

ROBERT A. CHASE, M.D.

President, November 1974 to July 1977

CHARLES F. SCHUMACHER, Ph.D.

Director, Department of Psychometrics

Lea & Febiger • *Philadelphia 1978*

First Edition 1971

Library of Congress Cataloging in Publication Data

Hubbard, John Perry, 1903–
 Measuring medical education.

 Includes index.
 1. Medicine—Examinations. 2. National Board of
Medical Examiners. I. Title. [DNLM: 1. Education,
Medical. 2. Educational measurement. 3. Medicine—
Examination questions. W18 H875ma]
R834.5.H8 1978   610'.76   77-19174
ISBN 0-8121-0625-3

Published in Great Britain by Henry Kimpton Publishers, London

Printed in the United States of America

Print number: 3   2   1

Preface

This second edition of *Measuring Medical Education* results from the extensive changes that have taken place in the policies and procedures of the National Board of Medical Examiners since the first edition appeared in 1971. Whether under its own responsibility or in cooperation with other agencies, the Board's services have greatly expanded as it creates, scores, analyzes and reports objective examinations. The results of those examinations provide valid and reliable measurements of the knowledge and clinical competence of medical students, physicians in training and physicians in practice. The measurements of individuals, who are the product of the educational system, may be analyzed and studied collectively for classes of students and groups of physicians at varying points of development, thereby yielding objective assessments of the effectiveness of the educational system. Evaluation of the product thus provides evaluation of the process.

We do not wish to imply that objective measurements obtained by examinations are necessarily the most appropriate or best method of evaluating medical students or medical education. The continuous assessment of individual students by their own faculties has advantages that cannot be superseded by formal, sporadic extramural examinations, no matter how good the latter may be. At the institutional level, formal accreditation of medical schools has long been well established as a function of the Association of American Medical Colleges and the American Medical Association through a joint Liaison Committee on Medical Education, representatives of which periodically conduct on-site surveys, studies of educational facilities and face-to-face interviews with faculty and students.

Objective measurements of medical knowledge and competence of individual students, as described in the following chapters, have, however, introduced a new and useful dimension of the educational system. With due recognition of the variability in the raw material of medical education, that is, the students as they enter medical school, their medical knowledge and competence as measured at intervals along the educational path provide assessments, limited though they may be, of the educational process.

These assessments and the methods of obtaining them as described in the following chapters are the outgrowth of twenty-five years of experience in the application of the science of educational measurement to the science of medicine. As the experience grew, so too did calls upon the services of the National Board and so also did the staff—but always with an effort to maintain a balance between those with backgrounds in medicine and medical education and those with backgrounds in psychometrics. This second edition, therefore, is the product of a highly competent, experienced staff, the senior members of which are listed in Appendix A. Although all deserve recognition for their roles in the procedures and accomplishments described in the following pages, special recognition is due to those who have participated in the authorship of certain sections and chapters of this second edition.

Dr. Edithe J. Levit, President of the National Board of Medical Examiners, although not identified as author of any section or chapter of this book, shares in all that made the volume possible. Her creative imagination, tireless energy and persuasive influence within the staff and with external agencies played a major part in the innovative developments that have kept the Board's services in the forefront of evaluation of American medical education. It was Dr. Levit who, soon after the acceptance of multiple-choice testing techniques at graduate as well as undergraduate levels, was instrumental in introducing the objective measurements of clinical competence that characterized the Board's Part III examinations and were adopted by American specialty boards. As Secretary of the Board's Committee on Goals and Priorities, she was the principal architect of the report to which she gave the title *Evaluation in the Continuum of Medical Education*,* a report which gained prompt attention from coast to coast. As is the case with any vigorous report, it was met with criticism in some quarters, but in all quarters the strength of its recommendations was recognized. There emerged a clearer concept of the sequential, lifelong educational continuum (a term this report did much to popularize) and the need for a parallel evaluation continuum.

Dr. Robert A. Chase, in his position as President of the Board from November 1974 to July 1977, was responsible for the continuing momentum of the Board's activities at a time when increasing pressures were arising from the public and from within medicine itself to provide assurance that those providing health services were adequately qualified to do so. Public accountability became the watchword and the National Board's role in producing qualifying examinations was further expanded and even became mandated, whether wisely or not, in

---

*Evaluation in the Continuum of Medical Education. Report of the Committee on Goals and Priorities of the National Board of Medical Examiners (William D. Mayer, Chairman). National Board of Medical Examiners, Philadelphia, 1973.

requirements written into federal law (The Health Professions Educational Assistance Act of 1976). Dr. Chase's account of the position of the National Board during this critical period is clearly set forth in his summary chapter, Chapter 11: The National Board and the Public Interest: Pertinent Areas of Activity.

Dr. David E. Smith, Vice-President and Director of the Board's Department of Undergraduate Evaluation, joined the staff with a background of experience in medical education as Professor and Chairman of the Department of Pathology at the University of Virginia followed by a period of staff responsibility for the American Board of Medical Specialties. He had become familiar with and a part of the policy making of the Board as a member of its Executive Committee for many years. He was, therefore, in an excellent position to guide the development and use of the Board's examinations in Parts I, II and III and the examinations derived therefrom (see Chapters 3, 4 and 8) and, more generally, in his capacity as Vice-President to bring his broad experience to bear upon the ongoing policies and activities of the Board.

Dr. William B. Kennedy, Co-Director of the Undergraduate Department, came to the National Board from his position as Associate Dean at the University of Pennsylvania School of Medicine, in which position he had been instrumental in persuading the faculty to accept the National Board examinations in lieu of a faculty-made multiple-choice examination. From this background, he was in an excellent position to work with the test committees for the Board's own examinations and to monitor the use of standardized test material for those agencies that depended upon this resource for the many derivative examinations described in Chapter 8. Because of his familiarity with the Board's extensive collection of examination questions as it stood the test of usage, he was the one who formulated the sample examination at Appendix B—one of the most popular features of the first edition of this volume.

Dr. Fred D. Burg, Vice-President and Director of the Department of Graduate and Continuing Medical Evaluation and formerly holding a joint appointment in the American Board of Pediatrics, became recognized as the National Board's most active and energetic link with evaluation of graduate and continuing medical education. In collaboration with the American Board of Medical Specialties, the individual specialty boards and the medical specialty societies, Dr. Burg and Dr. Bryce Templeton, then Co-Director of his department, extended the role of the National Board in evaluation of the continuum of medical education as described in Chapter 9.

Dr. Charles F. Schumacher, Director of the Department of Psychometrics, coming to the Board from the Research Division of the Association of American Medical Colleges, brought to the Board the needed strength in the science of educational measurement. During a period of rapid expansion, his unswerving adherence to the principles of psychometrics coupled with an innate sense of research kept progress tempered with realism. His chapters on scoring and analysis and on reliability, validity and standard setting (Chapters 5 and 6) are his most direct contributions to this volume, but his hand, and that of his Co-Director, Dr. Paul R. Kelley, are also to be found in all aspects of the Board's responsibility for maintaining the precision of its examinations.

Dr. Barbara J. Andrew, Director of the Board's Department of Research and Development, speaks for herself in Chapter 10 in describing the emphasis the Board has given and continues to give to research and development in educational measurement. This feature of the National Board, which began with its comparative studies of essay and multiple-choice examinations, continued through exploration of better ways to measure clinical competence and included studies in the relevance of individual test questions. Prompted by one of the prime recommendations of the Board's Committee on Goals and Priorities, the Department of Research and Development was set up within the staff to give focus and leadership to the continuing effort to find better ways to measure medical education at all levels.

Dr. Ethel Weinberg, Associate Director of the Department of Undergraduate Medical Evaluation, has served as Director of the Allied Health Professions Evaluation Programs, one of the activities of the National Board that was undertaken as this category of health professional came into national recognition. Accordingly, she has had special interest in examination validity and contributed substantially to its discussion in Chapter 6.

These then are the members of the staff upon whom I relied for an updating of the policies and procedures of the National Board of Medical Examiners as of 1977. But they are only a part of the total staff that is uniquely qualified in medical education and its evaluation and ably supported by dedicated managerial personnel. Working closely together, its members have become known and respected nationally and internationally for their leadership in meeting the ever-increasing demands for accurate and meaningful measurement of medical education. To each I am grateful for creating the substance from which this volume is derived.

Finally, although a publisher may not usually be given thanks for the part played in the preparation of a volume, I wish to express my appreciation for the skillful and understanding editing done by Mrs. Rosemary Pattison, our editor at Lea & Febiger and one-time member of the staff of the National Board of Medical Examiners.

Philadelphia   John P. Hubbard, M.D.

Contents

CHAPTER 1

■

The Evolution of Measurement and Evaluation

There have evolved on the American medical scene three distinctive functions on which the profession and the public rely for assurance that the educational system is producing the desired results: (1) evaluation of the individual who is the product of the system, (2) evaluation of the educational process and (3) evaluation of the institution responsible for the education. The first is intimately related to the sanction given by the profession or legal authority permitting (licensing) the individual to practice medicine. The second involves judgments about the effectiveness of the institution in achieving its educational objectives. The third calls upon the educational institution to show evidence that it is meeting specified criteria of established standards whether at the level of the medical school, the teaching hospital or, now, those additional agencies and organizations involved in continuing education.

Evaluation of the Individual

The Apprentice System

In colonial days and for some time thereafter in the United States, reliance upon the apprentice system, perhaps after some medical education abroad, was about all that there was to give the patient some sort of confidence in the knowledge and skills of the "doctor." We are inclined to disparage the apprentice system in the light of today's formal education and legal controls over the practice of medicine, but—with the current large numbers of students going through the educational system and with the resulting difficulties in providing for close association between the student and the master of the art and science of medicine—we might well give some thought to its values.

Genevieve Miller gives us a vivid example of the manner in which the student was evaluated and deemed competent to enter the practice of medicine in colonial America.[1] She cites a Virginia physician who penned the following certificate for his apprentice in 1775:

> These Presents will Inform All whom are Concern^d that Mr Cary Henry Hampton of the County of Pr William in the Colony of Virginia hath

Compleat[d] his Apprentisship to my Instruction in the Arts & Scienes [sic] of Anatomy, Chirurgery, Physic & Midwifery to all of which for the space of four years he hath been Studious & Diligent. He is well grounded in the teachings of Cheseldens Anatomy, Heisters Surgery, Cullens Materia Medica, Smellies Midwifery, the Works of our Masters Sydenham & Hippocrates which he hath read in the Latin tongue, as well as many other books of our Proffession and in the Instruction I have give to him at the beds of my Patients & elsewhere. So I repose my Confidence in his Knowledge & Reccommend him to all those who require his Skill & Services.
Given under my hand & seal this the first Day of Aug[t]. 1775
Andrew Robertson Doctor in Medicine

This document constituted young Hampton's "license" to practice. Its acquisition was far from casual. Legal indentures bound the medical student to his teacher just as craftsmen of all kinds were bound to their masters in the vocational training of the medieval guilds. In a Massachusetts indenture of 1734 the medical preceptor was obliged to provide meat, drink, washing and lodging for five years and four months while the obligation of the student was as follows:[1]

During all which said term the said apprentice his said master and mistress honestly and faithfully shall serve; their secrets keep close; their lawful and reasonable commands everywhere gladly do and perform. Damage to his said master and mistress he shall not willfully do; . . . Taverns nor alehouses he shall not frequent, or cards or dice, or any other unlawful games he shall not play. Fornication he shall not commit, nor matrimony contract with any person during said term. From his master's service he shall not at any time unlawfully absent himself, but in all things as a good, honest and faithful servant and apprentice shall bear and behave himself.

State Licensing Boards

It was inevitable that this very personal system, which obviously by its nature was limited in the number of young physicians that it could accommodate, would become increasingly inadequate. Quacks, charlatans and nostrum pushers were numerous and laws were needed for the protection of the public.

In 1760 the General Assembly of New York enacted legislation forbidding anyone to practice medicine or surgery in the city of New York who had not first been examined and approved by a board consisting of a member of the King's Council, the judges of the Supreme Court, the King's Attorney-General, the Mayor of the city of New York or by any three or more of them. As might be anticipated, such a board would be handicapped without the participation of physicians in the examination.

In New Jersey in 1772, the provincial medical society which had been formed in 1766 requested the government to set a licensing system for the province. Accordingly, the legislature and Governor William Franklin (son of Benjamin) adopted an act to regulate medical practice throughout New Jersey. This statute required that all those wishing to practice "Physic and Surgery" should be examined and approved by any two of the judges of the Supreme Court with the assistance of any persons they thought fit to aid in the examination. Thus was created the prototype of the later state boards of medical examiners. This auspicious beginning of an attempt to gain some control over the practice of medicine under state authority did not make much headway; most states delegated the licensing authority to the state medical societies.

Following the founding of the first American medical schools, a new problem arose for the evaluation of the individual for the practice of medicine. The College of Philadelphia (now the School of Medicine of the University of Pennsylvania) was founded in 1765; it was followed by King's College in 1768 (now the College of Physicians and Surgeons of Columbia University) and Harvard Medical School in 1782. As recounted by Shryock:[2]

> The problem of whether medical schools as well as societies could issue licenses first appeared in Massachusetts, where the second medical society was authorized in 1781 to examine candidates without reference to guild distinctions. The first men so examined—like most of the examiners—had been trained only by apprenticeships. After the Harvard Medical School was founded in 1783, however, the question arose: Should any further examination be required of its graduates?
>
> The medical society at first insisted on its right to pass on every man who desired certification—with or without a degree. Under pressure, however, a public examination was held of all candidates, and the Harvard M.D.s so outshone the others that licenses could not be long refused to such men. After 1803 *either* the Harvard diploma or examination by the society qualified a man for practice.

As medical schools developed, control over entry into the practice of medicine seemed promising. In nearly all states, examinations were required either within the schools or before state boards or societies. Unfortunately, however, the promise proved illusory. The prestige that accompanied the M.D. degree led to a proliferation of medical schools that varied in quality. Between 1810 and 1840, 26 schools were established, and between 1840 and 1875 an additional 47. Members of the faculty were paid by fees received from students and were tempted, therefore, to care more for the size of the class than the learning of the student. Bargain degrees could not easily be distinguished from those obtained from better schools; furthermore it was assumed by some that second-grade physicians were needed anyway to look after the poor.[2] The lowering of standards was hastened by the rapid expansion of the country westward. The need for physicians was great and the public was not particularly demanding of quality. For example, in Tennessee, as reported by Shryock,[2] there were, in 1850, 201 "physicians" of whom 35 were graduates of some sort of regular school; 42 said they had taken one course of lectures; 27 belonged to the cult of "Botanic and Steamers" while most of the others had received no instruction other than "reading, which for the most part was limited."

By the middle of the nineteenth century, it was apparent that steps had to be taken to bring order out of chaos. The awarding of licenses after examination by a legally constituted state board, begun so auspiciously in New Jersey in 1772, had been surrendered to medical societies and medical schools of variable standards. In 1846, the New York State Medical Society initiated a call for a national organization that would gain some control over the standards of medical education and the prevalent practice whereby professors licensed their own students—who provided them with fees for attending lectures. In response to the call from New York, the American Medical Association was founded at a meeting in Philadelphia in 1847.

With the support and urging of the AMA, the state boards of examiners gained strength and they in their turn moved toward national organization. In 1891, they founded the Confederation of State Medical Examining and Licensing Boards.

As stricter requirements for a state license developed, new problems arose for the practicing physician who sought to carry his medical license from one state to another. To meet this problem one state board might arrange reciprocity with another, thus accepting the standards of the second state. Among those states that agreed to recognize each other's licenses, a physician could move without the threat of repeating his licensing examinations. This trend led to the formation of the Confederation of Reciprocity which later (1913) merged with the Confederation of State Medical Examining and Licensing Boards to form the Federation of State Medical Boards.[3]

The system of reciprocity was, however, limited in effectiveness because of the variability of standards from state to state. Some states had reciprocity with some others, some with many, some with few. The physician who wanted to move to a state with which his home state did not have reciprocity had to face up to licensing examinations covering the general fields of medicine, examinations that he had passed upon completion of his formal medical education but which presented an awesome challenge years later.

Proposal for a National Board of Medical Examiners

In January 1902, well into the period characterized by Shryock as the age of medical reform, an editorial appeared in the *Journal of the American Medical Association* promoting the formation of a "national board of medical examiners."[4] It is probable that this editorial was written by William L. Rodman, who enlarged upon the proposition in a paper in the *Philadelphia Medical Journal* in May 1902 as follows:[5]

At the recent meeting in Washington City of the Committee of National Legislation representing the American Medical Association, the subject of reciprocity between the several states was very generally discussed, and considered practically impossible with so many states and territories, each with its own standard and no two alike. In some states there is no State Board of Examiners and the several counties of the states fix a standard. More than half of the states were represented at the conference, and the interchange of opinion was free. The committee appointed one year ago made a majority report through its secretary. Dr. Emil Amberg, advising against reciprocity, and in favor of a national board of examiners. The committee had, however, been working upon the hypothesis that such a board could be created and sustained by act of Congress. Letters read from Senator Burrows and others caused the committee to drop the idea of a National Board created by Act of Congress, as such legislation would certainly be unconstitutional and in conflict with the several states. The states are sovereign and cannot be coerced by the general government.

There is, however, nothing to prevent, or seriously in the way of, a voluntary National Board of Examiners, whose examinations shall be of such a character and high standard as to command the respect of the several states and cause them to issue a license to any one who has successfully passed such an examination. To fail to do so, as was said by Professor William H. Welch in the discussion, would make such state ridiculous. . . .

This plan has been unanimously endorsed by the delegates from the several states meeting with the committee on National Legislation and will be recommended to the House of Delegates at the coming meeting of the American Medical Association. It is to be hoped that it will be carefully considered and either it or a better plan at once inaugurated; as something should be done to encourage a higher and better medical education and to give in return something in the way of privileges and professional standing to those possessing it.

A second paper by Dr. Rodman, appearing a month later in the same journal, suggests that the voice of the state boards had been heard in opposition to his proposal.[6] He wrote: "There being a little misconception as to the exact purpose of a Voluntary National Board of Examiners, which I advocated at the April meeting of the Committee on National Legislation representing the American Medical Association, in the City of Washington, I will explain the plan more fully." He then proceeded to repeat the description of his proposal but with added emphasis on the importance of the autonomy of the state boards:

I would not have any one think me antagonistic to State Boards. On the contrary, it is my belief that they have done more than all other influences combined to elevate and make possible the present high standard of medical education. I feel, and have said on many former occasions, that every teacher in this country does better work now than he did before there were State Boards to examine the candidates whose diplomas he signed. Recognizing the good work done by State Boards, and believing them to be capable of doing even better work in the future, I would like to see a member of this Voluntary National Board a representative of the National Confederation of State Medical Examining and Licensing Boards. . . .

The national and state boards would thus work hand-in-hand.

Again Rodman noted that the plan had been unanimously endorsed by the delegates from the several states and that it would be recommended to the House of Delegates at the forthcoming meeting of the AMA. At this meeting in Saratoga Springs in June 1902, the proposal was formally introduced:[7]

The Secretary of the National Confederation of Medical Examining and Licensing Boards, was given the privilege of the floor and stated that a voluntary board of national examiners had been considered by the Confederation and a resolution not approving such a board had been adopted. Dr. William H. Welch then moved that a special committee of five be appointed by the President to consider the question of a national examining board for license to practice and of inter-state reciprocity, and that the above resolution from the Confederation of Examining Boards be also referred to this committee, the committee to report at the next year's meeting of the House of Delegates. In the minutes of the New Orleans' session in 1903, there is no mention of a report of the Legislative committee on a voluntary board of medical examiners.

No action having been taken by the House of Delegates at the Saratoga meeting, problems relating to reciprocity continued to mount as discontent with the existing order continued to develop. Various remedies were suggested, but the state boards were unable to solve these problems. The idea of a national board of medical examiners as a solution was again discussed in the *Journal of the American Medical Association* in 1906 by Dr. John M. Dodson, who, at that time, was dean of the Rush Medical College of the University of Chicago.[8] His logic was unassailable. He called attention to the inability of the state boards acting jointly to reach a consensus relating to minimal standards needed for licensure, and he spoke of the need for an outside, unprejudiced agency to perform this function. The acceptance of the examinations of this agency by the particular state boards would be entirely voluntary and, therefore, the survival of such a national board would depend upon its excellence. Again no action was taken. A further editorial appeared in the *Journal* in September 1914 proposing such a board, but the subject was not brought before the entire profession.

The following year (1915), the indomitable and persistent Dr. Rodman, undaunted by years of opposition and inaction and now President of the American Medical Association, included in his Presidential Address at the Annual Meeting on June 22, 1915, in San Francisco, an announcement of the fact that a National Board of Medical Examiners *had been* established, that its members *had been* appointed and that it would hold its first examination in Washington the following October.[9] He stated that:

> To meet a situation which, under our peculiar form of government, has resulted in hardships, and must, if continued, cause countless embarrassments, a National Board of Medical Examiners has been organized, and will hold its first examination in Washington in October. The character and scope of this examination will be such that no state ought to, and we believe none will, deny recognition, in the fullest sense, to those who pass it . . .
>
> All of us have in mind sad examples of able, even distinguished, general practitioners and specialists who, compelled to remove from one state to another, were estopped from practicing their profession . . .
>
> For many reasons, a national board with power to confirm a diploma carrying with it the unquestioned right to practice in any state—indeed to follow the flag—had always been desirable . . .
>
> It should be a simple matter to induce all of the states at once to recognize a national board whose only aim is to improve the existing situation.

Eight states agreed to accept the National Board's examination: Colorado, Idaho, Kentucky, Maryland, New Hampshire, North Carolina, North Dakota, and Vermont.

Shortly after the formation of the Board, two events occurred that affected its course significantly. One was the death of Dr. Rodman in March 1916, and the other was the entrance of the United States into World War I in 1917. Dr. Walter Bierring, representing the Federation of State Medical Boards, was elected to fill the unexpired term of Dr. Rodman, and Dr. William Rodman's son, Dr. J. Stewart Rodman, who was serving as assistant secretary, was named secretary. For the next forty years, the labors and advice of these two men proved to be of inestimable value.

The National Board held its first examination in October 1916 in Washington, D.C., using the facilities of the government hospitals there. The examination continued over a full week and included written papers, oral quizzes and practical demonstrations with patients and pathological specimens. There were 32 applicants, of whom 16 were considered qualified. Ten appeared and five passed.

The first meeting of the full Board was held in November 1916 at which time the educational standards of the Council on Medical Education of the AMA were made applicable to candidates for National Board examinations, with the additional requirement of at least one year of service in an acceptable hospital after graduation.

The requirements then became: (1) a diploma from a high school of good standing giving a four-year course, (2) a satisfactory college course in science, embracing physics, chemistry and biology, of not less than one year, (3) four years in a medical school of A grade and (4) at least one year of internship in an acceptable hospital.

The pace of the growth of the Board was slow at the outset, due in part to the entry of the United States into World War I. Shortly after the war was over and the Board had an opportunity to examine its progress, attention was immediately focused on the effectiveness of the examination. A commission composed of Col. Louis A. LaGarde and Dr. Walter L. Bierring was sent abroad in 1919 to study the operations and techniques of the qualifying boards in England, Scotland and France. The small delegation was well received; one who offered considerable help was Sir William Osler, then at Oxford.

Soon after this visit, there was a return visit from representatives of the national qualifying boards of England, Scotland and the Academy of Paris. As a result of this international exchange, Dr. Stewart Rodman proposed an examination following the pattern of the established procedures of the Triple Qualifying Board of Scotland and the Conjoint Examining Board of England.

The examinations were then set up as essay tests in the traditional basic medical sciences (Part I), and in the clinical-science subjects (Part II). A third part, Part III, was an oral "practical" examination. Part I was usually taken by students at the end of the second year of medical school and Part II toward the end of the fourth year. A year of internship was required for admission to Part III. Thus, as the student proceeded through his years of formal education and acquired an M.D. degree, he had the opportunity to qualify for a state license by taking and passing the three-part series of extramural examinations.

For the individual taking the examination, the point of critical importance was a passing mark. Although the examinee showed the natural tendency of students to strive for grades higher than the bare minimum for passing, the state licensing boards were really interested only in a record showing that the candidate had "passed the National Boards."* If he had passed, he could be given a license by "endorsement" of his National Board certificate without further examination; if he had failed, or if he had not taken National Boards, he must then take the examination of a state board of medical examiners. As an increasing number of states throughout the United States recognized the high standards of the National Board, its examinations became widely accepted as a minimum standard—to be sure a respectably high but nonetheless minimum standard—for the general practice of medicine.

Thus, there came into being a system unique to the United States: the admission of physicians to the practice of their profession at the conclusion of a formal education that has built into it a series of extramural examinations the results of which are regarded by official licensing authorities as an impartial, dependable and acceptable qualification for a license to practice.[10]

The close association that had been formed between the newly created National Board and the well-established qualifying boards of England and Scotland led to promising arrangements for at least some degree of reciprocity across the Atlantic. Successful performance on Part I of the British examinations was accepted for admission to Part II of the National Board examinations and vice versa. This was a step that brought much-needed gain to the prestige of the National Board in its early critical days and today might well be brought to mind in the light of current interests in international qualification for medical practice, as discussed in the 1976 conference of the National Board dealing with this very subject.[11]

The early pace of acceptance of National Board examinations by state boards would have been disappointing to its founder, Dr. William Rodman, who, as noted above, stated in his historic Presidential Address that: "It should be a simple matter to induce all of the states at once to recognize a national board whose only aim is to improve the existing situation." From the eight states that initially accepted the certificate of the National Board as qualification for the practice of medicine without further state examination, the count grew slowly at first and then increased to include 43 of the 48 states at the time of the Board's 25th anniversary in 1940. All state boards have accepted National Board certification at one time or another, but at no one time, not even today, do all states accept National Board examinations.

Introduction of Multiple-choice Testing

In the early 1950s, a change was introduced with effects more far-reaching than were appreciated at the time. Objective multiple-choice testing methods had come of age. It appeared timely to marry the science of medicine to the

---

*We recognize that there are many "national boards" of examiners. Throughout this volume we will, however, refer to the National Board of Medical Examiners as the Board or as the National Board and to its examinations as the National Boards. In doing so, we are merely following popular usage throughout the medical community. We would also note that the board is not, as its name suggests, an official governmental agency; it is incorporated as an independent, nonprofit organization. Further, it is not to be confused with the many boards of medical specialties.

emerging science of educational measurement. A study was undertaken with the cooperation of the Educational Testing Service to determine the applicability of multiple-choice testing methods to the field of medicine. After three years of deliberate, carefully designed experimentation, convincing evidence supported the conclusion that multiple-choice methods were superior to the time-honored essay methods for the purposes of the Board.[12,13]

Part I and Part II were converted to multiple-choice form. (Part III continued as an oral, bedside examination for another ten years until new techniques were developed for objective evaluation of clinical competence.) Each Part was reduced from three to two days, since two days of multiple-choice tests were found to provide a much more comprehensive examination than had the earlier three days of essay tests.

Part I included a total of about 800 to 1000 multiple-choice questions in the basic medical sciences equally divided among anatomy, biochemistry, microbiology, pathology, pharmacology and physiology. Additional questions have recently been added in the behavioral sciences, recognizing the increasing acceptance of behavioral science as a basic science in the medical-school curriculum. The time allowance was 12 hours during two successive days. Thus the students were required to respond to the questions at a rate averaging about 70 to 80 an hour. This rate would be expected to vary considerably during the examination depending upon the length and the problem-solving nature of the questions, but at this rate most medical students found the scheduled time sufficient without an undue sense of haste or pressure.

Part II was also scheduled for 12 hours with 800 to 1000 multiple-choice questions in the clinical sciences divided equally among internal medicine, obstetrics and gynecology, pediatrics, preventive medicine and public health, psychiatry and surgery.

The change to the multiple-choice form led to precise grades free of the subjective judgments of essay examiners. In essay-test days a single examiner wrote the questions and read the responses of thousands of candidates. He alone determined the grade for each examination on the basis of his independent judgment of the responses. In multiple-choice testing, the correct response for each question is determined as the question is created. The scoring becomes an objective count of the examinee's responses marked on an answer sheet. Furthermore, the responsibilities for the design of the examination, for the formulation of the questions and for the correctness of each question are placed upon committees of examiners; these examiners write the questions which are then reviewed, accepted, modified or rejected in outspoken, frank and free-swinging discussions in meetings of peers. For the Board's complete three-part series of examinations the number of examiners, serving on about 15 separate committees, is approximately 100. Their expert comprehension of the subject matter and their prominence both in their special fields and in the broader area of medical education are elements of prime importance in establishing and maintaining the high quality of National Board examinations.

The members of the test committees have a challenging experience as they meet together with the medical and psychometric members of the National Board staff. Most important, they bring back to their medical schools a deeper awareness of ways in which to develop and interpret objective examinations.

Evaluation of the Process

As increasing numbers of faculty members learned more about these examinations, medical schools themselves began to show a growing interest in the scores obtained by their students. The Board then began to receive requests to make its examinations available for whole classes irrespective of the individual student's interest in taking them as a qualification for a state license. Thus two categories of medical students emerged: those who elected to take the examinations as candidates for certification and those who were taking the examinations only as a requirement of the faculty. A new dimension had been created for evaluation of the educational process. Precise, reliable and useful data provided an additional measure of the effectiveness of the educational program of individual schools. Class scores for the basic-science subjects or the clinical-science subjects could be compared intramurally. Similar comparisons could be made with classes of students in other schools on a department-by-department basis, or for the basic-science subjects or the clinical-science subjects as a whole.

A subtle yet profound change in the role of the National Board began to appear gradually. No longer was the objective limited to a threshold examination for admission to the practice of medicine. The distribution of scores within a class, and the class averages, became matters of significance to the faculty as well as to the students. The scores could be used—and in many schools were used—to influence the standing of the student in his class. Mean scores of the class were studied by the faculty in relation to the curriculum in general and in detail. The examinations, having originated as an evaluation of the *product* of medical education, had become an instrument for the evaluation of the *process* of medical education.

The first comparative evaluation of medical schools based upon reliable measurements of student performance was published in 1954.[14] A more extensive description of the purposes and methods of constructing, scoring and analyzing multiple-choice examinations in medicine, and their value for group comparisons, was published in 1961.[15]

The role of the National Board at the level of undergraduate medical education therefore became twofold: (1) to measure as precisely as possible the achievements of individual students, providing thereby a means by which a physician may be accepted as qualified for the practice of medicine, and (2) to offer medical schools reliable comparisons of the effectiveness of teaching in individual schools. The Board has repeatedly emphasized its conviction that its role is to measure the results and effectiveness of the educational system, not to direct it. Undeniably, there is an overlapping relationship between the educational system and the examination system. Close as that relationship is, however, the Board is on the side of the examination system. Its position is unique as a testing agency drawing its competence from highly selected leaders of the nation's medical faculty who meet together free from the responsibilities and problems of curriculum design in their own schools and departments, and whose task is to construct the instruments whereby the effectiveness of the educational system may be assessed.

This task gains added importance in the light of the pressures arising both from the public and from the medical profession for increased numbers of physicians to meet what is often spoken of as the "crisis" in the nation's health manpower. New schools are being established, existing schools are pressing toward enrollments three or four times the number thought to be maximal only a few years ago, and curricula are being cut in length. The examiners of the National Board are aware of their challenging responsibility to provide a valid basis for stability and continuing quality at a time of widespread pressures for quantity.

Accreditation of the Institution

The distinction between evaluation of the individual and accreditation of the institution must be kept clearly in mind as two closely related but separate responsibilities and functions. When reliable extramural examinations became available for medical school faculties to use for their students as comprehensive examinations or on a departmental basis as guides to the evaluation of the educational process as described above, the question of the applicability of the examination results for evaluation of the institution arose. How did one school compare with another on the basis of group scores? Which were the ten best schools based on performance on National Board examinations? Which schools ranked lowest? These questions were not unfamiliar to the National Board in the early days of objective multiple-choice examinations.

It has, however, been a firmly and consistently held policy of the National Board that specific examination scores would be reported only: (1) to the individual examinee, (2) to the medical school and (3) at the request of the individual to a state board of medical examiners or other agency as he might request. As the popularity of the examinations increased and as more and more medical school faculties found them useful as an internal index of the knowledge and problem-solving abilities of the students, analyses of the group scores of school classes were reported to medical schools so that the faculty could judge the performance of the class in comparison with other schools or on a department-by-department basis within the school. In these reports, results were in terms of comparison with mean scores or the standing of the student class in a frequency distribution of all participating medical schools, with the identification of the schools held strictly confidential. For further discussion of the values, the uses and the misuses of extramural examinations for internal use of medical schools, and the ways in which examination results have more recently been reported to medical schools, see Chapter 7.

On the American scene, however, evaluation of the institution does not rest on the results of examinations and the measurements that may be derived therefrom. Evaluation of the institution is based upon quite a different system, and the appropriate term here is *accreditation*.

When the landmark Flexner report of 1910[16] threw its glaring spotlight on the extreme variability of the quality of medical education throughout the United States and the "enormous over-production of uneducated and ill trained medical practitioners," strong impetus was given to the inspection of medical schools by the AMA's Council on Medical Education, started a few years earlier in 1906. Schools were ranked A, B or C. The class C schools soon disappeared.

Some class B schools survived for some years, but they too no longer exist.

In 1942, the Association of American Medical Colleges (AAMC) joined the AMA Council on Medical Education in establishing the Liaison Committee on Medical Education (LCME). The LCME then became the authoritative agency with responsibility for establishing the criteria for accreditation of medical schools and, by means of periodic visits of inspection, for determining if the criteria have been met. These criteria have been most recently reviewed, updated and published by the LCME in a statement entitled "Accreditation of Schools of Medicine: Policy Documents and Guidelines."[17]

The criteria governing decisions about accreditation require assessments made through on-site visitations and resulting assessment of the school's "constellation of resources in relation to the total student enrollment." This constellation of resources includes such essential features as the duration (a minimum of 32 months) of planned required and elective activities, administration and governance, number and quality of the faculty, finances and facilities, all in relation to the school's stated goals and objectives. Each year a report on the accreditation of medical schools is published in the AMA's Annual Report on Medical Education in the United States.[18]

As medical education has extended to include not only the "undergraduate education" of the student in medical school but also the graduate (postgraduate) education of the physician in hospital internship and residency and the continuing education of the physician throughout his professional career, the concept of the continuum of medical education has become a reality. Complex interrelationships of responsible agencies have been formalized within a Coordinating Council on Medical Education (CCME) having representation from the AMA, the AAMC, the American Board of Medical Specialties, the American Hospital Association and the Council of Medical Specialty Societies. This Council, created in 1972 with its carefully established representation, is in a position to coordinate the responsibilities for the accreditation of institutions involved in the emerging continuum of medical education.

The National Board of Medical Examiners on the other hand, although deeply involved in evaluation in the continuum of medical education as described in following chapters, has no role in the function of accreditation of institutions. It has endeavored to make its position on this point altogether clear in the statement in the recently published report on "Evaluation in the Continuum of Medical Education":[19] (1) that the National Board of Medical Examiners recognizes that its role is solely in the realm of evaluation of individual competence, and (2) that the responsibility for setting standards of professional performance, certification of specialty competence and legal licensure should continue to reside with those organizations presently having such responsibilities.

Expansion of the Board's Role in Evaluation

With the increasing acceptance of the reliability, validity and excellence of the Board's examinations and examination services, it was called upon increasingly to extend its services in the measurement of medical education and evaluation of qualification for the practice of medicine. This expansion, described more fully in the Annual Reports, is shown graphically in Table 1.

Table 1. Extension of Examination Services: 1955–1975

Examination Services	1915–1955	1960	1965	1970	1975
Type/Purpose of Exam	Certifying Exams for Licensure ──→				
		Educational Achievement Exams (I and II) ─────────────────────→			
		Custom-made Exams from NBME Pool ────────────────────────→			
			Specialty Board Written Exams ─────────────→		
				Residency In-training Exams ──→	
				Self-assessment/Continuing Education Exams ──→	
Relationships with External Agencies	Individual State Licensing Boards ──→				
		Medical Schools/Departments ───────────────────────────→			
		ECFMG—FSMB—MCC ───────────────────────────────→			
			Specialty Boards and Specialty Societies ──→		
Educational Level	Undergraduate/Internship ──→				
		Graduate Medical Education ────────────────────────────→			
				Continuing Medical Education ──→	
Health Profession	Medical Students/Physicians ───→				
				Physician's Assistants ──→	

The Board first took on the role of a service agency in the early 1950s when it began to provide its examinations to medical schools for their own use in assessing educational achievement. Since these examinations were essentially derived from the regular examinations of the Board, this service function involved providing a ready-made product plus scoring and reporting of results.

Soon thereafter, as organized medicine addressed the confused situation resulting from the influx of foreign medical graduates into this country, the Educational Commission for Foreign Medical Graduates (ECFMG) was established, and the National Board was asked to participate in the development of a screening examination to be given to foreign graduates who sought internships and residencies in this country. This proposal represented a new departure in the Board's traditional function since it involved the development of a qualifying examination for a purpose other than licensure. After careful deliberation by the National Board, satisfactory agreement between the two groups was established and the ECFMG gave its first examination in March 1958.

This decision denoted yet another important change with respect to the type of examination services provided in that, for the first time, the National Board was engaged in developing "custom-made" examinations constructed entirely from the National Board pool of calibrated test questions. A further extension of this service came about with the Board's decision, in the mid-1960s, to collaborate with The Federation of State Medical Boards of the United States, Inc. (FSMB) in developing the Federation Licensing Examination (FLEX) which is also based upon test material drawn from the National Board's pool of questions. A similar service has been provided to the Medical Council of Canada (MCC) in the creation of its examinations for licensure. In the latter two instances, while continuing in a relationship to licensing boards, the National Board assumed an examination service function quite different from its traditional role as an independent certifying agency.

Examination Services to Specialty Boards and Societies

In 1961, the decision to provide assistance to the American Board of Pediatrics marked the beginning of a new and different service role which did not involve the use of the National Board's own test material. For the first time, the Board was asked to provide consultative, professional and administrative services with the explicit understanding that the specialty board itself would have the final responsibility for and control over the design, development and use of the examination.

Other specialty boards followed the example of the Board of Pediatrics and, for the first time, the National Board was now involved in the evaluation process beyond the internship level. Providing assistance to specialty boards marked the beginning of the National Board's involvement in evaluation in graduate medical education. As at the undergraduate and licensure levels, the services of the National Board were soon sought by institutions and agencies for purposes other than certification, e.g., the development of in-training examinations for residents.

Beginning in 1967, with its decision to work with the American College of Physicians in the development of its first self-assessment examination, the National Board moved into an entirely new and different area of activity: providing examination services that were designed to serve the needs of individual physicians who were voluntarily assuming responsibility for their own continuing education. They were not utilized by institutions and agencies accountable to the public for assuring professional competence. This new activity marked the Board's first involvement in the evaluation process beyond the formal period of undergraduate and graduate medical education, and into the period of continuing education throughout the physician's career.

Certifying Examinations for Physician's Assistants

Throughout all of these developments and rapidly expanding activities, from its establishment in 1915 until 1972, the Board's services had been provided only to those organizations and agencies concerned with the education, licensure and certification of physicians. In 1972, arising from a recommendation during the early deliberation of the Board's Committee on Goals and Priorities[19] and following extensive study and consultation with a number of national professional organizations, the National Board undertook the responsibility for developing a certifying examination for a newly emerging category of health professional, namely, the assistant to the primary-care physician. The argument for moving into this new field was straightforward: The National Board has established skill and experience in evaluating the competence of the physician; the physician's assistant is doing a part of the job of the physician; this new health professional should be subjected to an appropriate measurement of competence.

The first National Certifying Examination for Primary Care Physician's Assistants was administered in 1973.* In 1975, sponsorship of the examination was assumed by the newly formed National Commission on the Certification of Physician's Assistants. The Commission is an independent certifying agency the composition of which includes the National Board, the American Medical Association, the American Academy of Physician's Assistants and twelve other professional groups. The Commission is responsible for the certification process, including the establishment of eligibility requirements and standards of performance. The National Board of Medical Examiners continues to develop and administer the examination under contract with the Commission.

The certifying examination is designed to measure the knowledge and skills necessary for performance as a physician's assistant. Test materials in medicine, obstetrics-gynecology, pediatrics and surgery are designed to assess competence in data gathering, analysis and interpretation, management (including technical and emergency procedures) and counseling.

The 1975 examination consisted of a half day devoted to assessment by multiple-choice questions and a half day to assessment by means of patient

---

* The work was supported by the Bureau of Health Manpower of the National Institution of Health, The Robert Wood Johnson Foundation and the W. K. Kellogg Foundation.

Table 2.   NBME Examination Services: 1950–1976

management problems. In addition, each candidate's abilities in performing physical examinations of five principal systems were evaluated by examiners using specially prepared checklists. The checklists were scored and included in the pass/fail decision for the examination.

All materials in the certifying examination are created by test committees composed of teachers of physician's assistants, practicing physician's assistants and physicians. The materials are selected in relation to specific health care functions identified by an Advisory Committee on Physician's Assistants.

Growth in Examination Services

The expanding dimensions of the National Board's role in evaluation at all levels of medical education is reflected in the growth pattern of examination services over the twenty-five years from 1950 to 1976. Table 2 shows this growth pattern in terms of the cumulative number of individuals examined, as well as the subtotal for the several categories of examination services.

The dramatic increase in examination services between 1960 and 1970, as documented in the foregoing discussion, reflects the multiple new dimensions of the Board's role in evaluation. On the other hand, the growth from 1970 to the present is primarily related to an increasing number of examinations provided in each of the major categories, and especially in examination services for specialty boards and societies.

The data for 1976 show that the examinations in Parts I, II and III, once the total program of the Board, now account for only about 25 per cent of all examination services. Examinations such as FLEX and ECFMG, which are based entirely on the Board's test material, account for an additional 32 per cent of examination services. Thus, with the addition of examinations provided directly to medical schools, National Board examination material was the basis for testing about 72 per cent of all examinees last year. Examination services for specialty boards and societies account for the remaining 28 per cent of those tested during 1976.

References

1. Miller, G.: A physician in 1776. JAMA, 236:26, 1976.
2. Shryock, R. H.: Medical Licensing in America, 1950–1965. The Johns Hopkins Press, Baltimore, 1967.
3. Derbyshire, R. C.: Medical Licensure and Discipline in the United States. The Johns Hopkins Press, Baltimore, 1969.
4. Editorial: National board of medical examiners. JAMA, 38:108, 1902.
5. Rodman, W. L.: Voluntary board of national examiners. Phila. Med. J., 9:837, 1902.
6. Rodman, W. L.: The proposed national examining board, a second paper. Phila. Med. J., 9:1012, 1902.
7. Bierring, W. S.: First twenty-five years—a few memoranda and memories. Read before the National Board of Medical Examiners. New York, June 12, 1940.
8. Dodson, J. M.: National examining boards. JAMA, 47:877, 1906.
9. Rodman, W. L.: Work of American Medical Association. JAMA, 64:2107, 1915.
10. Hubbard J. P.: The role of examining boards in medical education and in qualification for clinical practice. J. Med. Educ., 36:94, 1961.
11. Annual Conference of the National Board of Medical Examiners: An International View of Qualification for the Practice of Medicine. Philadelphia, March 1976.
12. Cowles, J. T. and Hubbard, J. P.: A comparative study of essay and objective examinations for medical students. J. Med. Educ., 27(Part 2):14, 1952.

13. Cowles, J. T. and Hubbard, J. P.: Validity and reliability of the new objective tests. J. Med. Educ., 29(6):30, 1954.
14. Hubbard, J. P. and Cowles, J. T.: A comparative study of student performance in medical schools using National Board examinations. J. Med. Educ., 29(7):27, 1954.
15. Hubbard, J. P. and Clemans, W. V.: Multiple-choice Examinations in Medicine. Lea & Febiger, Philadelphia, 1961.
16. Flexner, A.: Medical education in the United States and Canada. Bulletin #4, Carnegie Foundation for the Advancement for Teaching, New York, 1910. Reprinted by the Arno Press and the New York Times, New York, 1972.
17. Accreditation of Schools of Medicine: Policy Documents and Guidelines. Liaison Committee on Medical Education of the Council on Medical Education of the American Medical Association and the Executive Council, Association of American Medical Colleges, 1976.
18. Medical Education in the United States, 1975–1976. JAMA, 236:2949, 1976.
19. Evaluation in the Continuum of Medical Education. Report of the Committee on Goals and Priorities of the National Board of Medical Examiners (William D. Mayer, Chairman). National Board of Medical Examiners, Philadelphia, 1973.

CHAPTER 2

■

Test Committees and their Tasks in Creating Objective Examinations

The Committee Method

One of the most outstanding features of the National Board's method of creating multiple-choice examinations is test construction by carefully selected committees. These committees are made up of subject-matter specialists who meet together with the test specialists of the staff. Creative writing—and the preparation of good multiple-choice questions is one of the most exacting forms of creative writing—is not usually done best by committees. In this instance, however, experience has shown that two heads are better than one and several heads better than two.

As mentioned in the previous chapter, the Board's corps of examiners is drawn from among the leaders of medicine and medical education in the United States and Canada. These men and women know medical education because they are doing it. As medical education changes they are intimately aware of the changes, because they themselves are involved in them.

Each of the major subjects of Part I and Part II is the responsibility of a separate committee that usually numbers six to eight individuals who are experts in their respective fields. Thus biochemists construct the test questions in their field for Part I; pediatricians are responsible for the questions in pediatrics in Part II. Part III, on the other hand, is a multidisciplinary examination without orientation along departmental lines and is, therefore, the responsibility of multidisciplinary committees.

This corps of examiners currently includes about 110 individuals with broad geographic representation among medical schools. They serve with a rotating membership, usually for a period of four years. A committee of six to eight has been found to be about optimal. In a smaller committee, the work falls heavily on few individuals; in a large committee, there is apt to be so much discussion that the work of the committee may suffer. With a committee of six to eight individuals each serving four years, one or two members rotate off each year to be replaced by carefully chosen successors; there is therefore a constant infusion of fresh talent to take over from those who may have become weary of the task.

The criteria for the selection of a committee member are few but essential: (1) prominence in the field so that he or she can take a place at the committee table as a peer of those already on the committee, (2) commitment to medical education and its evaluation, (3) awareness of the rapid changes in the medical educational environment. It is not necessary that the newly appointed committee member have specialized experience with test techniques. The role is that of a subject-matter specialist who will soon become familiar with the do's and dont's of test construction as the questions submitted for committee approval are subjected to the frank comments of colleagues. Even experienced examiners may fall into the trap of ambiguity in wording test items or may find that, for other reasons, their test items (test questions) are not acceptable to colleagues on the committee. They learn that every word must have precise meaning. As Lindquist has pointed out, "Few other words are read with such critical attention to implied and expressed meaning as those used in test items."[1]

Outline of Examinations

The committee begins with formulation of an outline of the intended content of the test. The purpose of this outline is to make certain that all of the important aspects of a discipline or subject are sampled and that a specified number of questions is included for each category. This procedure not only ensures a comprehensive coverage but also allows for weighting of subject matter, so that more questions can be allocated to one category and fewer to another as judged appropriate by the committee. This outline is reviewed and revised annually to keep the test in step with changing emphases in teaching and with new concepts in medicine.

The outline is drawn up in the way that the examiners agree is best suited to their particular subject. The National Board's test committee for physiology designed an outline which, as might be expected, reflects the physiologists' viewpoint related to body functions. The outline for pediatrics was, on the other hand, approached from a very different point of view, as illustrated below:

Physiology Outline

1. Fluid and electrolyte balance, renal mechanisms
   a. Excretory functions, filtration, excretion, secretion, reabsorption, circulation, renin
   b. Body fluids, blood volume, blood-brain barrier, cerebrospinal fluid, acid-base balance, electrolytes

2. Cardiovascular physiology
   a. Cardiac electrophysiology
   b. Cardiac cycle, mechanics and output
   c. Hemodynamics
   d. Circulation in specific organs

    e. Cardiovascular regulation
    f. Capillary exchange and lymph

3. Metabolism: energy balance, starvation, temperature regulation, fever, hypothermia, muscular exercise

4. Endocrinology and reproduction
    a. Neuroendocrinology
    b. Regulation of metabolism: fluids and electrolytes, protein, fat, carbohydrates
    c. Reproductive processes and their regulations

5. Gastrointestinal functions: digestion, hepatic mechanisms, secretions, motility, endocrine and neural control

6. Respiratory and pulmonary functions
    a. Mechanics of breathing
    b. Pulmonary gas exchange
    c. Blood gas transport and tissue gas exchange
    d. Regulation of respiration

7. General and cellular physiology

8. Nervous system and special senses
    a. Autonomic and somatic motor mechanisms
    b. Central integrative processes covering consciousness and other complex behavior
    c. General properties of sensory mechanisms and somatic sensation
    d. Vision, audition and other special senses

Pediatrics Outline

1. Newborn: prenatal, premature, term
2. Growth and development: physical, behavioral, emotional; congenital anomalies
3. Nutrition, metabolic and genetic disorders: breast feeding, artificial feeding, deficiency diseases, inborn genetic disorders including inborn errors of metabolism, fluid and electrolytes
4. Infectious diseases and immunology: viral, bacterial, parasitic, protozoan, fungal, other; immunology, including immunizations
5. Systemic diseases, including neoplasms: alimentary, respiratory, cardiovascular, genitourinary, hematologic, neuromuscular, endocrine
6. Therapeutics: choice of drugs, dosage, common procedures
7. Accidents: poisoning, other
8. Legal medicine

For each of the test outlines a limited number of categories of subject matter has been found to be advisable. If there are too few categories, important topics may be omitted; a large number of categories may be difficult to handle, since then there may not be enough items adequately to test each category.

Having decided upon the categories needed to cover the subject adequately, the committee determines the per cent of the total test to be allocated to each category. One category may be allocated 20 per cent of the total number of test questions; another, considered less important, may be given 5 per cent. In a test of 150 items, about the average total for one of the major subjects, a category with less than 3 per cent, or about five items, is too small to have any real meaning.

The category outline has two functions. First, it serves to remind the test committee of the areas of the subject that they have agreed upon as important. Second, the outline is distributed to all those registered for the examination so that they may have advance notice of the general content of the test; at the same time they are given examples of the form of the test questions (see Chapter 3) so that they can become thoroughly familiar with the test technique in advance and during the examination can concentrate on the content. The percentage distribution of the questions and the resulting weighting of the categories are not, however, made known to the examinees.

Comprehensive Multidisciplinary Examinations

The Part I and Part II examinations are each scheduled for two consecutive days with six or six and one-half hours of testing time for each day. The twelve or thirteen hours for each Part are equally divided among the major subjects, i.e., approximately two hours each. The number of multiple-choice questions that examinees can be expected to handle during the allocated time varies considerably, depending upon the length of individual questions and the time required for thoughtful attention to problems presented in varying degrees of complexity (see Chapter 3). The average for the National Board's Parts I and II is usually about 75 to 80 questions per hour. Thus, each of the separate committees is responsible for introducing into the test approximately 140 to 150 multiple-choice questions. If a particular test is designed to contain a considerable number of time-consuming questions, these may be put together into a separate section of the examination with fewer questions per hour, or, in distributing questions throughout the tests, time-consuming questions may be balanced with others that require less time so that time is available for all. After all, the purpose is to test the knowledge of the examinee and his ability to apply his knowledge to the problem in hand, not to see how many questions he can answer in a given period of time.

That the examination system may keep closely in step with the changing nature of the educational system, Parts I and II are set up and scored as total multidisciplinary examinations; there is no identification of individual test questions according to subject-matter areas. The grade for each Part is based on the total number of questions answered correctly rather than on an average of the grades for the component subjects. Irrespective of performance in individual subjects, the examinee passes the Part by answering correctly a sufficient number of questions to yield a passing score on the test as a whole (see Chapter 5). Individual subject grades have continued, however, to be reported for each of the traditional subjects for Part I and Part II, to meet the requirements of individual state licensing boards calling for specified grades in individual subjects. Also, despite protestations to the contrary, medical schools and medical students continue to manifest interest in grades in the separate subjects.

To adjust to the changing and variable patterns of the curriculum, eligibility requirements for Part I and Part II are flexible; any student regularly enrolled in any approved medical school in the United States or Canada may register for either Part I or Part II at any regularly scheduled administration. The student need not wait until completion of the second year to take Part I or until his fourth year to take Part II, as had earlier been required. Thus, emphasis is placed upon acquisition of knowledge and competence rather than upon completion of predetermined periods of time.

Students find that the multidisciplinary nature of the total examination and of individual questions is closely suited to their experience during medical school. The grading procedure is in keeping with the use of elective time now prevalent in medical schools. Since passing the examination is dependent only on the percentage of questions answered correctly in the total examination, students can and do compensate for weakness in certain areas with better-than-average knowledge of other areas in which they have special interest and perhaps have had elective work.

The Construction of the Test

The preparation of each National Board examination takes approximately one year. Each committee member writes a number of questions in accordance with the outline and with the assignment determined by the committee itself. This assignment may require an individual qualified in a particular subspecialty to write all of the questions in this area of special competence; alternatively, it may be considered preferable for the required number of questions in each category to be divided among the committee members.

One of the firmly held principles of the committee method of constructing National Board examinations is that members of the committee will be responsible for any test item they submit. It is not necessary that they write the questions themselves; they may enlist the help of colleagues in the same department or consultants from other departments. Each committee member must, however, approve the content and the wording of each question submitted since, irrespective of the authorship, the question will be regarded as that member's contribution for review by the committee.

The National Board does not favor the custom, sometimes encountered in other boards or examination committees, whereby multiple-choice questions are solicited from members of the board who do not meet with an examination committee and have no further responsibility for the examination. The justification for this "mail-order" method of obtaining test questions is a desire to involve the board members or others in the specialty in the preparation of the examination. This may be good for the board member but it is not good for test construction. Too many items are received in unacceptable form and with unacceptable content, and the author of a question that may have been aimed at an important target is not there to explain the purpose of the question and to help put it into an acceptable form.

To make the submitted questions fairly uniform in style, special forms are provided to each committee member. After new items are received on these forms, they are duplicated and assembled in a draft that includes not only the newly written questions but also previously used test questions selected from the National Board's pool. Each of the examinations of Parts I, II and III, therefore, may contain questions tested by previous use. Both new and previously used questions are distributed to all members of the committee who are asked to study each item carefully and to determine whether it appears satisfactory as written, whether changes are indicated or whether the question is inappropriate and should be discarded. This study and criticism of individual questions are done as homework before the committee meets for a two-day session of frank, critical, around-the-table discussion of each individual item.

At these two-day committee meetings, each member of the committee is asked for comments about each question based upon review prior to the meeting. If the question is approved by committee consensus, with or without modification, it is then marked for final draft of the test. If it duplicates another question or needs revision, it is set aside for future use. If it is judged as too difficult, too easy, inappropriate, ambiguous or for other reasons unacceptable, it is discarded altogether. Those who participate in this exercise are impressed with the value of group dynamics in arriving at final decision for acceptance or rejection of an individual test question. A far more penetrating critique arises here than through independent and individual judgment.

At this stage of their review by the committee, the questions are arranged according to categories of subject matter so that the committee members may see the content of the examination category by category. Later, when selection of the questions for final copy has been completed, the questions are rearranged and mixed with questions of the same item type from other subjects so that, in taking the test, the examinee encounters items of one type at one time. Then, following an appropriate set of instructions, the examinee passes along to the next type of question, and the next, in an orderly manner. At this point, care is taken to assure that the correct responses are distributed randomly. For example, there should not be a long series in which D is the correct response, followed by another series in which B is the correct response.

As the questions are approved, discarded or set aside, consideration is given to the categories of subject matter and to the types of items. The number of items in each category is made to conform to the subject-matter outline. Attention is also given to the number of items of any one type; five is the number usually considered the minimum to justify a separate type of item under separate instructions. The selected questions are then typed and duplicated as an initial test draft that is reviewed by a committee of the chairmen of the several committees. Again, duplications, inconsistencies or other faults in individual questions or in the test as a whole are noted and eliminated. Thus there are three separate occasions when each single test item is subjected to critical review not only by members of the test committees but also by the highly skilled and experienced test editors of the Board: (1) in the homework prior to the meeting, (2) in the committee's review of the new material to be introduced into the test and (3) in the final test draft.

Admittedly, the creation of multiple-choice examinations by committees of experts is time consuming and laborious, but free and frank discussion among colleagues produces results that cannot be achieved by any other method. Despite the exceptional qualifications of the examiners, the experience of the

National Board reveals that, on the average, about one-third of the questions as originally written need revision. About one-third are discarded as too difficult, unimportant, controversial or for other reasons not appropriate for the examination. Only about one-third of the questions originally submitted are accepted with little or no change. Consequently, confidence can be placed in the fact that each question has been thoroughly worked over and agreed upon as appropriate in content and difficulty, free from ambiguity, accurately and concisely written and representative of important aspects of the subject.

Reference

1. Lindquist, E. F. (Ed.): *Educational Measurement.* American Council on Education, Washington, 1957.

CHAPTER 3

■

Types of Multiple-choice Questions

Three Basic Types of Questions

Twenty-five years ago, after the National Board of Medical Examiners had converted its written examinations from essay to multiple-choice questions in cooperation with the Educational Testing Service (ETS), various types of multiple-choice questions used successfully by the ETS were adopted by the National Board. It became apparent, however, that test construction for the National Board was quite different from test construction for the ETS. The National Board, dealing with examination content specifically in the field of medicine, was relying upon panels of examiners drawn from medical school faculties who wrote the test questions themselves at home and then worked together with the Board's test experts at the conference table; most of these examiners had had little or no previous experience in creating multiple-choice questions. Certain complicated types of questions, although they had worked well in the hands of the ETS, were viewed by the National Board examiners as contrived and more likely to assess an examinee's test-taking ability than his knowledge of medicine.

After several years of experience with this relationship between the examiners who wrote the questions and the test experts at the National Board, and as a result of careful studies of the comparative values of different types of questions, the National Board cut back in the variety of types of questions that had been used in earlier days in multiple-choice examinations in medicine, as described by Hubbard and Clemans.[1] The Board now uses three basic types of multiple-choice questions. Each type has several variations and, as described in Chapter 4, new testing techniques have been introduced to provide objective measurements of clinical competence.

One-best-response Type (Item Type A)

This is the traditional and most frequently used type of multiple-choice item. (In the language of multiple-choice testing, it is customary to speak of test items rather than test questions since they are frequently presented in the form of statements rather than questions.) This type of item consists of a stem (e.g., a statement, question, case history, situation, chart, graph or picture) followed by a series of four or five suggested answers for a question or completions for a statement. The suggested answers (completions) other than the one correct choice are called distracters.

A series of five choices (one correct answer plus four distracters) is preferred to a series of four choices. In a five-choice item, an individual knowing nothing about the subject matter has a one-out-of-five (20 per cent) chance of choosing the correct response by random guessing; in a four-choice item, his chances increase to 25 per cent by random guessing.

In this type of item (item type A), the instructions to the examinee emphasize the importance of selecting the "one best response" from among those offered. The item usually has a comparative sense: one procedure is clearly the best out of the five choices; one diagnosis is the best among those given; one value is the most accurate response to a required calculation. In the broad field of medicine, however, contrasts are seldom sharply defined as black and white, but are apt to be varying shades of gray. In answering these questions, therefore, the examinee is instructed to look for the *best* or *most appropriate* choice and to discard others that may appear plausible but are in fact less applicable.

Here is a straightforward example of the one-best-response type:

Item 1.* The most effective prophylactic agent for the prevention of recurrences of rheumatic fever is
    (A)   acetylsalicylic acid
    (B)   para-aminobenzoic acid
    (C)   adrenocorticotropic hormone
    (D)* penicillin
    (E)   cortisone

In this example the stem might have been written as a question: "Which of the following is the most effective prophylactic agent for the prevention of recurrences of rheumatic fever?" There is little advantage in an incomplete statement over a question, but the incomplete statement is sometimes preferred because it can often be expressed in a simpler way with fewer words.

In the above example, D is the correct response and those designated as A, B, C and E are incorrect responses, or the "distracters." In the preparation of multiple-choice questions, the development of effective distracters is one of the most difficult parts of the examiner's task. Each distracter should be a plausible answer and should fit into the context of the problem at hand. Inconsequential or implausible wrong answers should be strictly avoided. Any distracter that is obviously wrong weakens the test. If, for example, two out of five choices are so patently wrong as to present no problem to any of the examinees, the correct response becomes a one-out-of-three choice with a 33 per cent chance of a correct response by random guessing among the remaining options.

One of the criticisms often made of the multiple-choice type of test arises from having the correct response included among the answers offered so that the examinees may be reminded of something they might not have thought of

---

* All items are numbered consecutively throughout the text. Correct responses are identified by an asterisk.

without seeing it spelled out. It is not, however, necessary to name the correct response among the given choices. The above item could be written as follows:

Item 2. The most effective prophylactic agent for the prevention of recurrences of rheumatic fever is
    (A) acetylsalicylic acid
    (B) para-aminobenzoic acid
    (C) adrenocorticotropic hormone
    (D) cortisone
    (E)* none of the above

In this manner the examinees must search their minds for the prophylactic agent most effective in the prevention of recurrence of rheumatic fever without having this agent, penicillin, suggested to them by finding it as one of the possible choices.

Again, using the above item as an example, it might be written as follows:

Item 3. The most effective prophylactic agent for the prevention of recurrences of rheumatic fever is
    (A) acetylsalicylic acid
    (B) para-aminobenzoic acid
    (C)* penicillin
    (D) cortisone
    (E) none of the above

In this version, the "none of the above" response is incorrect and the correct response becomes C. It should be made clear to the examinee that the "none of the above" choice may sometimes be correct and sometimes incorrect. Also, when "none of the above" is used as the fifth choice, meticulous care must be taken to be sure that each choice is unequivocally correct or incorrect.

Another variant of the completion type of item is the negative form: All but one of the choices are applicable and the examinee is asked to select the one which does not apply, or applies least, or is an exception in some way. The following is an item of this type:

Item 4. Active immunization is available against each of the following diseases EXCEPT
    (A) tuberculosis
    (B) smallpox
    (C) poliomyelitis
    (D)* malaria
    (E) yellow fever

For a correct response to this item, the examinee must know that agents are available for active immunization against all of the diseases mentioned except malaria. This "each of the following EXCEPT," however, requires a switch from positive to negative thinking; this may throw the examinee off the track to the extent that an incorrect response might indicate a failure to follow the technique of the test rather than a true lack of knowledge of the subject. To avoid this possible difficulty, test items with negative stems may be placed together in a separate section of the test with special instructions calling attention to their negative form; alternately, the same subject matter may be stated positively by using the multiple true-false type of item (see page 32).

"All of the above" should not be used as a fifth distracter. Among a set of four choices followed by "all of the above" as the fifth option, it is likely that an examinee would recognize at least one as clearly incorrect. Therefore, not only this but the "all of the above" response can be eliminated, leaving a one-out-of-three choice rather than the intended one-out-of-five. Furthermore, if the examinee knows that any two of "the above" are correct then "all of the above" *must* be the correct answer since any two correct responses among "the above" leave no other choice for *one best* response.

The best one-out-of-five type of test item may follow, either singly or in sets, the presentation of a case history or other situation presenting a problem that can be as complex as seems appropriate to the examiner. In presenting case histories or other problem situations, a clear and concise style is urged. The objective is to give the examinee all the necessary information—but *only* the information truly necessary to make the correct response out of the choices offered. Fulsome descriptions with literary embellishments serve only to use up the examinee's time unnecessarily.

To probe several aspects of the examinee's knowledge related to a case history or problem situation, two or more multiple-choice items may follow a single stem (e.g., case history). Care should then be taken to avoid interdependence of the items, so that an incorrect response to one item does not lead to incorrect responses in all of the others. For example, the first question following a complicated case history might require the examinee to make a diagnosis. If a second item dealing with confirming laboratory procedures or therapy then follows, the examinee is in double jeopardy if the right diagnosis has not been made in answering the first question.

The following case history describes a patient with hemophilia, but the word "hemophilia" does not appear anywhere in the question. The examinee must, however, know about hemophilia in order to respond correctly to the three mutually independent questions that follow the case history.

A 14-year-old boy is admitted to the hospital with a nosebleed which followed slight trauma and which has persisted for four hours despite nasal packing. He has had repeated nosebleeds since early childhood. He had spontaneous hematuria on one occasion, and has ankylosis of both knees and the left elbow as a consequence of hemorrhage into these joints following injury. A maternal uncle was also a bleeder, but his mother, father, and two sisters have not had abnormal bleeding.

He has a blood-soaked pack in his nose and ankylosis of both knees and his left elbow. His spleen is not palpable. There is no evident lymphadenopathy; no petechiae or telangiectases are seen. The following laboratory data are reported: hemoglobin 13 gm per 100 ml; erythrocyte count 4,500,000 per cu mm; leukocyte count 12,000 per cu mm; differential count normal; platelets 460,000 per cu mm; urine shows no protein, red blood cells, or other abnormalities in the sediment.

Item 5. Which of the following tests is most likely to show an abnormality?
 (A) Tourniquet test
 (B) Bleeding time
 (C)* Clotting time
 (D) Clot reaction
 (E) Bone-marrow examination

Item 6. An abnormality would be expected in
 (A) the one-stage prothrombin time
 (B)* the thromboplastin consumption test
 (C) plasma fibrinogen content
 (D) platelet fragility
 (E) none of the above

Item 7. The most efficacious of the following therapeutic procedures would be
 (A) local applications of thrombin-soaked packs to the nose
 (B) intravenous administration of a suspension of fresh, normal platelets in saline
 (C)* intravenous administration of fresh plasma
 (D) intravenous administration of vitamin K
 (E) intravenous administration of fibrinogen and calcium gluconate

Other examples of the one-best-choice form of item, illustrating the various ways in which this type can be used for both relatively short statements or questions and more complicated case histories and problem situations, are shown in Appendix B.

*The Matching Type (Item Types B and C)**

Items of a somewhat different nature may be used effectively to test knowledge of entities that may or may not be closely related. These items are particularly useful when dealing with the actions and uses of closely related drugs or the distinguishing signs or symptoms of similar diseases. A list of lettered headings is followed by a list of numbered words or phrases. For each numbered word or phrase, the examinee is required to select the one heading most closely related to it. Each heading can be used once, more than once, or not at all in the set.

In item type B, the leading list of headings may have varying numbers of entries; lists of five are preferred. Any number of items may be attached to the leading list. Care should be taken not to include items that are extremely easy or that deal with trivia merely in an attempt to get extra mileage out of the headings.

---

*Correct responses are indicated by the letter in parentheses.

Items 8 to 11 are examples of matching type B:

    (A) Hypertrophy of the left ventricle
    (B) Cor pulmonale
    (C) Mitral and aortic stenosis
    (D) Subpulmonic stenosis
    (E) Congestive failure without cardiac enlargement

Item 8.   Long-standing silicosis (B)

Item 9.   Constrictive pericarditis (E)

Item 10. Rheumatic heart disease (C)

Item 11. Systemic hypertension (A)

The leading list may have "none of the above" as an entry. Thus the candidate is challenged to think of possible associations other than those stated in the list. However, even more than with the use of "none of the above" in item type A, care must be taken to be sure that the association keyed as the correct response is unquestionably correct and that the numbered item could not be rightly associated with any other choice.

In another form of matching item, designated as type C, the examinee is directed to select the A response if the word or phrase is associated with A only, B if the word or phrase is associated with B only, C if the word or phrase is associated with both A and B, or D if the word or phrase is associated with neither A nor B. The following is an example:

    (A) *Plasmodium vivax* malaria
    (B) *Plasmodium falciparum* malaria
    (C) Both
    (D) Neither

Item 12. A combination of primaquine and chloroquine is the treatment of choice for an acute attack (A)

Item 13. Clinical attacks are suppressed by ingestion of chloroquine once a week while in an endemic area (C)

Item 14. Infection is prevented by ingestion of chloroquine once a week (D)

In the use of matching items, there is a temptation to add too many responses to a single stem. In the above example, three score points are involved in differentiating the features of *Plasmodium vivax* malaria and *Plasmodium falciparum* malaria. Many more items could have been included relatively easily. Therefore the examiner, especially when required to write a large number of items, should keep in mind the relative importance of the subject matter and the number of score points which a set of items of this type will contribute to the total test.

Multiple True-false (Item Types K and X)

Multiple true-false items consist of a stem followed by four or five true or false statements. The stem may be in the form of a question, a statement, a case history or clinical data presented in pictorial fashion as indicated in the sample test in Appendix B. When properly written, the multiple true-false question tests in depth the candidate's knowledge or understanding of several aspects of a disease, a process or procedure. Each of the statements or completions offered as possibilities must be unequivocally true or false, in contrast to the A type of item in which partially correct alternatives may be used as distracters. This type of question must be written so that no two alternatives are mutually exclusive, since the candidate is expected to consider the possibility that all of the choices may be correct.

One form of multiple true-false item, designated by the National Board as item type K, is characterized by a code that permits only one mark on the answer sheet and thus enables consistency of scoring to be maintained so that units can be summed throughout the examination with equal weight, irrespective of the item type. This feature is important when subscores are to be derived from interdisciplinary comprehensive examinations such as Part I or Part II of the National Boards.

In item type K, the examinee is directed to select the A response if 1, 2 and 3 are correct; B if 1 and 3 are correct; C if 2 and 4 are correct; D if only 4 is correct; and E if all four are correct. In the following example 1 and 3 are correct; the correct response is therefore B.

Item 15. A child suffering from an acute exacerbation of rheumatic fever usually has
(1) an elevated erythrocyte sedimentation rate
(2) a prolonged P-R interval on the electrocardiogram
(3) an elevated antistreptolysin-O titer
(4) subcutaneous nodules

Instructions for item type K are given in detail at the beginning of any section in which this item type occurs in the test; the code is also shown in abbreviated form at the top of every page where items of this type appear, as follows:

Directions Summarized				
A	B	C	D	E
1,2,3 only	1,3 only	2,4 only	4 only	All are correct

While partial knowledge is not automatically credited in scoring the K type (as opposed to one feature of the X type, see below), partial knowledge can be applied in guiding the examinee into the correct responses, and thus full credit, for a K-type item. If the examinee is certain that one (any one) of the four responses is correct, the number of possible correct lettered choices is reduced from five to three. Similarly if one is certain that one (any one) response is incorrect, the number of possible correct lettered choices is reduced to only two. A combination of any two such certainties usually yields the correct single answer, or at worst reduces choices to no more than two. For example, if one is certain that 2 is correct and 4 is incorrect, the answer can only be A. Equal certainty that both 1 and 4 are correct makes E the only possible answer. While some may consider this to be "testmanship," is it so different from the process one may apply in sorting out choices in arriving at a clinical diagnosis? In any event, experience has shown that examinees learn to handle the intricacies of the K type of item without great difficulty.

In another form of multiple true-false type, the X type, the examinee is instructed to respond separately to each of four or five choices so that any combination of rights or wrongs, from all wrong to all right, may be permitted. The above example of item type K (Item 15) would read exactly the same if it were presented as item type X. The instructions to the candidate would, however, read as follows:

You are to respond YES or NO to each of the four alternatives, bearing in mind that all, some or none of the alternatives may be correct.

For full credit for this item, the candidates would have to answer YES to 1 and 3 and NO to 2 and 4. Partial credit would be given for responses partially correct for the set, such as YES to 1 only or to 3 only (see example examination at Appendix B).

Studies undertaken by the National Board to compare the effectiveness and reliability of these two item types show that there is no significant difference in the rank order of the examinees when multiple true-false questions are set up in the form of item type K or item type X.

Pictorial, Tabulated and Graphic Material

A single picture, roentgenogram, graph or table may be presented and a set of questions developed to deal with it. Sets of two or more closely related pictures also may be used, followed by a series of questions requiring the candidate to utilize all of the visual material in choosing his answers.

In the simplest use of pictorial material, the names of disorders, lesions or other entities are given in the questions and the examinee is required only to match each one with the proper illustration. More is required of the examinee, however, if each question provides a brief clinical history, summary of laboratory data or suggested therapy. He is then required to interpret the illustration and to recognize a relationship existing between the information given and one of the illustrations. Questions accompanying graphs and charts may require the candidate to interpret the data and make certain deductions about them.

Pictorial material should clearly illustrate the point in question; it should not deal with trivia. Each question should be designed so that the examinee must refer to the visual material to arrive at the correct answer. When sets of illustrations are used and items call for a matching process, unintentional cluing (for example, a roentgenogram of a child in a series of roentgenograms where the identification of a child would give the examinee an obvious clue) is to be avoided.

For reproduction of roentgenograms or for pictorial material in color, the original transparency, that is, the original roentgenogram or 35-mm slide, provides the best quality. Glossy prints or lantern slides of roentgenograms or color prints result in less-than-satisfactory reproduction in the test booklet.

A good example of tabulated material to challenge candidates in depth in the understanding of clinical situations is shown below:

	Plasma Level mg/100 ml	Renal Clearance ml/minute	PAH Clearance ml/minute
Drug A	5	135	620
	10	130	600
	20	133	610
Drug B	5	65	612
	10	70	618
	20	68	606
Drug C	5	600	596
	10	450	604
	20	350	601
Drug D	5	600	604
	10	450	432
	20	350	354
Drug E	5	25	593
	10	60	603
	20	120	598

The above table lists the rates of renal clearance of a number of drugs in relation to their concentrations in the plasma of a human subject. All values are corrected for binding to plasma protein. The last column represents the simultaneous clearance of p-aminohippurate (PAH) at a plasma concentration permitting extraction of virtually all of the PAH in one circulation through the kidney. To answer Questions 16 to 20, select for each question the letter designating the drug which best fits the conditions described.

Item 16. Filtered by the glomerulus; partially reabsorbed by the renal tubules by a passive process (B)

Item 17. Secreted by the renal tubules by a rate-limited active transport process (C)

Item 18. Filtered at the glomerulus without tubular reabsorption or secretion (A)

Item 19. Reabsorbed by the renal tubules by a rate-limited active transport system (E)

Item 20. Secreted by the tubules but limits its own excretion by decreasing renal blood flow (D)

Good use of questions based on a graph is illustrated in Questions 21 and 22.

The graph below shows incorporation of radioactive iron in erythrocytes of peripheral blood after an intravenous injection of radioactive iron citrate. Study this graph to answer Questions 21 and 22.

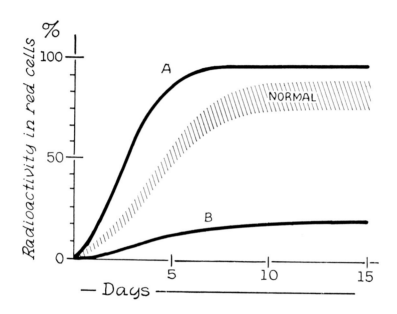

Item 21. A 40-year-old man has had prolonged gastrointestinal bleeding. He has an iron uptake as shown in curve A. This observation implies all of the following EXCEPT
    (A)   increased erythrocyte production
    (B)   iron deficiency
    (C)* saturated iron-binding protein
    (D)   reticulocytosis
    (E)   adequate serum folic acid concentration

Item 22. A 40-year-old man has normal erythroid blood values (hematocrit 45 per cent, hemoglobin 14.6 gm/100 ml, reticulocytes 1.0 per cent). His iron uptake is shown in curve B. These findings represent
    (A)   chronic glomerulonephritis
    (B)* hemochromatosis
    (C)   agnogenic myeloid metaplasia
    (D)   congestive splenomegaly
    (E)   low serum transferrin concentration

The sample examination at Appendix B includes examples of all types of questions currently used in National Board examinations and demonstrates the use of color plates, photographs, roentgenograms and electrocardiograms.

Checklist in Question Preparation

To aid the examiner in maintaining acceptable standards in the preparation of multiple-choice questions, the following checklist is offered. If an item does not satisfy each of these standards, it should be discarded or revised.

1. *Does the item deal with one or more important aspects of the subject?* Minutiae of medical knowledge are to be avoided.
2. *Does the item call for information that the examinee should know or be able to deduce without consulting a reference source?* Drug dosages, limits of normal values and other numerical data are to be included only if they deal with important information that should be within the daily working knowledge of the examinee.
3. *Is the item appropriate for the level of knowledge expected of the examinee?* Items that are too difficult or too easy cannot make effective discriminations among the examinees.
4. *Is the central problem stated clearly and accurately?* Wording that is ambiguous or fuzzy may mislead the examinee and destroy the validity of an item. All qualifications needed to provide a reasonable basis for an answer should be included.
5. *Have irrelevant clues to the correct response been avoided?* The most common clues are: the correct answer longer and more precise than the distracters, the use of common elements in stem and correct answer, inadvertent clues in grammatical construction, the use of "specific determiners" such as all, none, always and never.
6. *Is the item written with as few words as possible to make it clear and complete?* Unnecessary words increase reading time; the examination is intended to test medical knowledge, not reading speed.
7. *Is the item type the best one for the particular point or problem?* A topic difficult to test by one type of item may be probed without difficulty by another type.
8. *Is the item written in conformity with the format?* For example, in item type A, the choices (distracters) must be grammatically consistent with the main statement (the stem) and with each other.

Reference

1. Hubbard, J. P. and Clemans, W. V.: *Multiple-choice Examinations in Medicine.* Lea & Febiger, Philadelphia, 1961.

CHAPTER 4

■

Objective Evaluation of Clinical Competence

Ever since the beginning of National Board examinations, one part of the total procedure—a final Part III—has been included for the purpose of evaluating clinical competence. Before 1961, Part III was conducted as an oral bedside examination. After completing a history and physical examination of an assigned patient, the candidate was questioned by an examiner who was perhaps unfamiliar with the patient and who would, using the patient's chart, develop the examination along the lines of a quiz session that was an inadequate test of knowledge—the candidate's knowledge already having been more thoroughly tested in Parts I and II. The procedure would then be repeated at a second bedside, with another patient and another examiner. "Clinical competence" at the two bedsides might be, and often was, evaluated quite differently from examiner to examiner. The bedside evaluations were influenced by three variables: the examiner, the patient and the candidate. The increasingly apparent problem was how to control two variables, the examiner and the patient, in order to obtain a reliable measurement of the third variable, the one of critical interest, the candidate.

In 1959, the National Board undertook to analyze and define the clinical competence its Part III was intended to measure, and to devise testing techniques permitting objective, valid and reliable assessments of clinical competence as thus defined.[1,2] A two-year study was initiated with the cooperation of the American Institute of Research and its Director, Dr. John Flanagan, who had successfully developed objective methods for measuring skills of airplane pilots—another critical area of human responsibility.[3-5]*

Definition of Clinical Competence

The first step in this research project was to obtain a definition of clinical competence and skill at the level of the internship and hospital residency, as

*The National Board gratefully acknowledges a generous research grant from the Rockefeller Foundation in support of this project.

the young physician with his M.D. degree begins to assume independent responsibility for the care of patients. The method used was "the critical incident technique."[4] By interview and by mail questionnaires, senior physicians and residents, all of whom had direct responsibility for supervision of interns, were asked to record clinical situations (incidents) in which they had personally observed interns exhibiting, in their judgment, good clinical practice on the one hand and conspicuously poor clinical practice on the other. A total of 3300 incidents was collected from approximately 600 physicians. These incidents were divided about equally between "good" and "poor" practice. A review of these records provides an interesting—and also disturbing—description of actual behavior during internship. Among the most frequently reported examples of good clinical practice were: taking a history thoroughly and performing a physical examination in a systematic way, accurately recognizing the patient's condition from observation of clinical signs, withholding decision about diagnosis until all needed information was available, correctly suspecting an obscure diagnosis despite obvious symptoms and signs of another condition, and taking appropriate emergency action when indicated.

In contrast, the most frequently recorded examples of poor or inappropriate clinical practice were: failing to consider other than the most obvious causes of symptoms and signs, making a diagnosis with inadequate information and prescribing medication with inadequate indication.

The information resulting from the 3300 incidents was reduced to manageable proportions; the incidents were summarized individually, grouped and classified. They fell into nine major areas of clinical performance, with subheadings as follows:

1. History:
   A. Obtaining information from patient
   B. Obtaining information from other sources
   C. Using judgment
2. Physical Examination:
   A. Performing thorough physical examination
   B. Noting manifest signs
   C. Using appropriate technique
3. Tests and Procedures:
   A. Utilizing appropriate tests and procedures
   B. Modifying test methods correctly
   C. Modifying tests to meet the patient's needs
   D. Interpreting test results
4. Diagnostic Acumen:
   A. Recognizing causes
   B. Exploring condition thoroughly
   C. Arriving at a reasonable differential diagnosis
5. Treatment:
   A. Instituting the appropriate type of treatment
   B. Deciding on the immediacy of the need for therapy
   C. Judging the appropriate extent of treatment

6. Judgment and Skill in Implementing Care:
   A. Making necessary preparations
   B. Using correct methods and procedures
   C. Performing manual techniques properly
   D. Adapting method to special procedure
7. Continuing Care:
   A. Following patient's progress
   B. Modifying treatment appropriately
   C. Planning effective follow-up care
8. Physician-patient Relationship:
   A. Establishing rapport with the patient
   B. Relieving tensions
   C. Improving patient cooperation
9. Responsibilities as a Physician:
   A. For the welfare of the patient
   B. For the hospital
   C. For the health of the community
   D. For the medical profession

These nine major areas with their subdivisions, derived from factual information drawn from actual performance, constituted a well-documented answer to the question of *what* to test. The next step—and a formidable one—was to determine *how* to test designated skills and behavior of interns.

Many methods were explored: motion pictures, television, lantern-slide projection, various forms of the "tab test," and the technique developed by Rimoldi[6] to test diagnostic skills and reported by him in a series of papers.

At first these techniques were looked upon as possible supplements to, rather than substitutes for, the traditional bedside examination, long considered the ultimate in testing the competence of a physician. Therefore, in addition to the introduction of the new methods described below, an attempt was made to improve the reliability of the bedside examination. An evaluation form was carefully devised for an examiner to complete while watching the candidate taking a history and performing the physical examination. This form was also intended to standardize the oral examination directly related to the patient. As the candidate proceeded to a second patient and a second examiner, another copy of the same evaluation form was used. This method was used over a three-year period as a part of the examination; analysis of the results, however, indicated that it had not resolved the problem of the two variables examiner and patient, and did not therefore yield a reliable measurement of the third variable, the candidate. A study of the correlation between the independent evaluations of a single candidate made by the two examiners showed that agreement was still only at the chance level ($r = 0.25$ for a total of 10,000 examinations). The bedside examination was therefore discontinued after 1963.

The medium of motion pictures appeared to offer an objective method of testing many of the areas of clinical competence defined by the critical incidents study. In motion picture films a patient can be shown to all examinees at the same time. Questions about observable signs and features of the patient can then be asked in multiple-choice form. If sound accompanies the motion picture, a dialogue between physician and patient can be introduced to test the examinee's knowledge about skill in taking a clinical history and communicating with the patient. Auscultatory signs can be and have been included for testing purposes. In the experience of the National Board, however, the use of motion pictures, with or without sound, has failed to yield tests meeting the Board's high standards for certification examinations. Unquestionably motion pictures have gained a firm place in the educational system for purposes of teaching, but it is doubtful that they will be continued as a feature of National Board examinations in the same form in which they were introduced in 1961. It is more likely that motion pictures will be supplanted by other methods as computer technology advances and is coupled with projection capabilities for pictorial material and possibly linked to videotape or even to television.

Programmed Testing of Patient Management Problems (PMP)

A new and different testing method was devised and introduced by the National Board for the first time in 1961 to test aspects of clinical competence dealing with the ability to identify, to resolve and to manage patient problems.[1,2] This method simulates a realistic clinical situation in which the physician must face the dynamic challenge of a sick or injured patient. As in real life, the examinee is confronted with a patient about whom brief but carefully selected information is presented. This information must be studied and decisions reached about appropriate action. Laboratory studies and diagnostic procedures may be required; decisions about therapy and management are called for. In the test booklet, a list of possible procedures immediately follows the description of a patient. Some of these procedures are correct and mandatory for the proper management of the patient; others are incorrect or contraindicated. The examinee is not told how many procedures or courses of action are considered correct; the task is to select those considered indicated at this point in time.

On the front page of each test booklet instructions are given in detail. These can be found reproduced in the sample examination in Appendix B (page 170).

A sample problem illustrating the procedure to be followed is given on the back cover of each test book (see Fig. 1). The examinee is instructed to proceed with this sample problem in order to become familiar with the technique before turning to the test material itself. In this oversimplified problem, a brief paragraph describes a patient brought to the emergency room of the hospital in coma. From the information given, any intern would recognize the coma as due to diabetes. The first problem for this patient then offers six courses of action calling for immediate decision. Three of these choices (1, 3 and 4) constitute proper management at this point; selection of these three and only these three choices leads to a perfect score for this portion of the problem.

Figure 2 shows the answer blocks for choices 1 through 6 with the special pen having been applied to choices 3, 4 and 6. Choices 3 and 4 are correct procedures. The examinee has decided to catheterize the patient to test the

SAMPLE PATIENT

A 40-year-old comatose man with known diabetes mellitus is admitted to the hospital. There is no obvious evidence of trauma. On palpation, the eyeballs are soft. The skin is dry. Kussmaul's breathing is noted and the breath has an acetone odor. Temperature is 36.7 C (98.1 F) rectally; blood pressure is 100/70 mm Hg; the pulse is regular at a rate of 120/min. Examination of the chest shows labored respirations. The abdomen is soft; no masses are palpable. The liver and spleen are not enlarged. Deep tendon reflexes are hypoactive bilaterally.

SAMPLE PROBLEM S-1

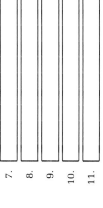

You would immediately: RESPONSE

1. Order a serum bicarbonate determination   1.

2. Order a serum calcium determination   2.

3. Order a blood glucose determination   3.

4. Order a urinalysis (catheterized specimen)   4.

5. Measure central venous pressure   5.

6. Perform a lumbar puncture   6.

SAMPLE PROBLEM S-2

You would now administer:

7. Digitalis   7.

8. Insulin   8.

9. Morphine   9.

10. Nikethamide (Coramine)   10.

11. An intravenous infusion of 0.9% NaCl   11.

INSTRUCTIONS FOR SAMPLE PATIENT

1. Study the initial information given.

2. Read all of the courses of action given in Problem S-1. Then choose the first option that you consider pertinent and necessary and, with the special pen provided, develop the area in the identically numbered rectangle that corresponds to your choice (Care: apply pen carefully and lightly). Proceed in a similar manner to any other options you may select.

3. After you have completed Problem S-1, bearing in mind the additional information resulting from your choice(s), proceed in a similar manner with Problem S-2.

4. In this simplified example of a patient in a diabetic coma, the correct courses of action in Problem S-1 are 1, 3, and 4; in Problem S-2, the correct courses of action are 8 and 11.

5. In this sample, as well as in the actual examination, responses are obtained for incorrect as well as correct courses of action.

6. For these sample problems only, you may now develop the areas in all of the rectangles to see the results of other choices.

Fig. 1.

SAMPLE PROBLEM S-1

You would immediately: RESPONSE

    1. Order a serum bicarbonate determination   1. [   ]

    2. Order a serum calcium determination   2. [   ]

    3. Order a blood glucose determination   3. [750 mg/100 ml *]

    4. Order a urinalysis (catheterized specimen) 4. [Glucose 4+; acetone 4+ *]

    5. Measure central venous pressure   5. [   ]

    6. Perform a lumbar puncture   6. [Scheduled *]

Fig. 2.

SAMPLE PROBLEM S-2

You would now administer:

    7. Digitalis   7. [Ordered *]

    8. Insulin   8. [Ordered *]

    9. Morphine   9. [   ]

   10. Nikethamide (Coramine)   10. [   ]

   11. An intravenous infusion of 0.9% NaCl   11. [   ]

Fig. 3.

urine, and the urine is found to contain large amounts of sugar and acetone, characteristic of the condition with which the candidate is dealing. If the candidate did not recognize diabetes as the cause of the patient's coma and selected choice 6—to perform a lumbar puncture—the erasure for this choice would reveal the word "scheduled." Thus, in very realistic fashion, the situation simulates that with which an intern might be confronted when the decisions are entirely his own with no senior physicians to advise him. He makes his own decisions and he obtains the results of his actions.

Having made his decisions for the immediate steps to be undertaken for this patient, the candidate then proceeds to the second portion of the problem. Figure 3 shows the answer blocks with items 7 and 8 having been selected by the examinee.

Developing Linear Patient Management Problems (PMP)

Examiners responsible for constructing patient management problems will find that the task is somewhat more complex than the creation of typical multiple-choice questions. At the National Board, an eight-step approach has been developed to aid in constructing patient management problems. Although the eight steps may seem rather simplistic, experience has shown that familiarity with these steps enhances the probability of achieving a patient management simulation of high quality.

Identify Problem and Correct Etiology

The examiner should determine on the basis of a variety of factors what the appropriate problem for evaluation by the PMP technique should be. Obviously, the problem should be related to the group of examinees being evaluated. In general, good problems for testing are those dependent upon the individual being able to gather appropriate data in a discriminating fashion and to differentiate among two to five plausible etiologies aside from that which is actually causing the patient's problem.

Write Differential Diagnosis

All etiologies that should be considered along with the correct one should be considered by the author of the PMP. By doing so the author then has reference points of other possible diagnoses that can be used to broaden the base of information included in the statement of the problem.

Determine Types of Tasks to be Simulated

Generally these tasks can be divided into three major categories: gathering data, assessing data and management.

Data Gathering. The patient management problem is designed primarily to assess an individual's ability to gather data appropriately. There are at least four subsets of data-gathering tasks: (1) history points, (2) physical examination activities, (3) noninvasive laboratory studies and (4) invasive laboratory studies.

In general, one or more of these subcategories can be used as a basis for the construction of a component part of each patient management problem. The experience of the National Board has been that, when patient management problems are designed to evaluate history taking and physical examination, data-gathering skills are least discriminatory.

Assessing Data. Skills in assessing data within patient management problems are somewhat limited. One approach has been to create a list of potential diagnoses that the examinees should consider at different points through a problem. One of the major problems with such a strategy is that the various diagnoses listed within a problem tend to clue the examinees into potentially identifying the cause of the problem which they might not have considered on their own.

Management. Generally, management tasks are evaluated most effectively toward the end of a patient management problem, since once a candidate begins to manage the patient there is a tendency for the problem to branch in a variety of directions. This can be confusing to the candidate and, therefore, it is generally wise to place the management section of a PMP as the last component of each case. There are at least three forms of management problems: (1) immediate (in terms of an acute emergency), (2) day-to-day and (3) follow-up management.

Determine Sequence of Tasks to be Evaluated

Depending on the particular problem and etiology, the order of task assessment will be variable. Therefore, it is suggested that examiners outline the order in which they would like to approach the assessment of the examinee's ability to deal with the various tasks listed above.

Identify the Situation

One of the most crucial components of the patient management problem is the initial descriptive paragraph, called the lead-in stem. Within this paragraph, the examinee is placed within the simulation. It is essential that the examiner identify for the examinee the following points: (1) What is the role of the candidate (e.g., consultant, primary care physician, surgeon)? (2) When does the problem take place? When is the patient seen (the time of day, if necessary the time of year)? (3) Where is the problem being presented (emergency room, office, hospital ward, etc.)?

Unless these three areas of who, when and where are carefully delineated, the examinee may be confused and have difficulty in participating within the simulation.

Write the Stem

A carefully constructed, concise stem dealing with the presenting problem as well as the above identification points is important to place the examinee within the appropriate milieu for the evaluation and management of the patient. Authors at times tend to write extensive stems which become distracting to the candidate. As can be seen in the sample on page 171, a concise stem gives the important elements of the history and physical examination.

Write the Problem

It is at this point that the examiner is placed in the position of having to identify appropriate options for all correct and incorrect diagnoses. Incorrect diagnoses fall into two major categories: those that are appropriate to consider as part of the differential diagnosis and those that should be excluded on the basis of important information received by the examinee. In constructing each of the various options for each of the various sections of patient management, the dichotomy between these two types of diagnosis is essential to keep in mind in order to determine the studies which should be ordered. The available choices may include studies that would be considered appropriate to eliminate an incorrect differential possibility; unless these are included, the validity of the problem tends to be diminished. Also, inappropriate choices for an inappropriate diagnosis, one that should have been eliminated on the basis of previously determined information, should be included.

Review for Cluing

Once a patient management problem has been constructed in relationship to the above-recommended steps, it is important that the examiner review the problem against each of the various appropriate and inappropriate diagnostic possibilities considered. The examiner should look for cluing between one problem and another which would allow an examinee either to backtrack and derive the correct solution or to find himself on a path overly directed toward the appropriate approach to the overall management of the patient.

Scoring Patient Management Problems (PMP)

The scoring of patient management problems gives credit for correct decisions and penalties for sins of omission and commission. Each of the several hundred choices, or courses of action, offered in the test is classified in one of three categories: (1) it must be done for the well-being of the patient; (2) it should definitely not be done and, if done, would be a serious error in judgment that might be harmful to the patient; and (3) it is relatively unimportant, i.e., a procedure that might or might not be done, depending upon local conditions and customs. Each examinee is given a "handicap score" equal to the total number of items coded as definitely incorrect. Each time the examinee selects an incorrect choice, one point is subtracted from this score; each time he selects a correct choice, one point is added. Thus, his total score on this test is the number of correct decisions he has made, i.e., the number of indicated procedures he has selected plus the number of incorrect procedures he has avoided. The choices in the equivocal middle ground receive no score.

The programmed testing method is quite different from the usual multiple-choice technique in which the candidate is offered a number of choices and instructed to select one best response. Here, he is offered a number of choices and required to use his best judgment in selecting all those, and only those, he considers important for the management of the patient. Usually, as in a practical situation on a hospital ward, he recognizes a number of actions that should definitely be done and other actions that should definitely not be done. His responses are therefore interrelated. If he is on the right track, he makes a number of correct decisions from among the available choices; then, by his erasures, he gains the information necessary for the proper management of the patient in the next problem and in the next set of choices. If he starts off on the wrong track in this programmed test, he may compound his mistakes as he proceeds and becomes increasingly dismayed as he learns from his erasures the error of his ways. If he discovers that he is on the wrong track, however, he has a chance to change his course and to make additional choices, although he cannot undo the errors that he has already committed—again a situation rather true to life.

Since in this testing technique, as in the use of the more traditional type of multiple-choice examinations, a panel of experts has determined the rightness or wrongness of each choice or course of action offered to the examinee, accurate and detailed statistical analyses are equally applicable. The essential criterion of test reliability will be dealt with in Chapter 6. Here it suffices to say that the reliability of the programmed testing section of Part III is generally at the level of .80 to .85,* which compares favorably to a section of equal length in Part I or Part II despite the fact that, in the desire to simulate real-life situations, interrelated responses are included within each problem and between one problem and the next. This interdependency has the effect of decreasing the number of points upon which the test score is built and also affects the accuracy of measurement of the reliability of the test.

This programmed testing of patient management problems has also been studied to determine the extent to which it is in fact measuring something different from that which has already been measured in the comprehensive examinations in the basic medical sciences (Part I) and the clinical sciences (Part II). Unless significant differences could be found, this portion of the examination would have added nothing to the assessments of the candidates already made. Correlations were, therefore, calculated between Part II and the PMP section of Part III; the correlations ranged from .34 to .48. These correlations, positive yet moderate, reflect the degree of correlation that would be expected between medical knowledge and additional elements of clinical competence inevitably based upon medical knowledge but representing skills that are to a degree independent of factual knowledge. If these correlations were high, they would have indicated that the patient management problems were measuring the attributes already thoroughly measured, and the test would be superfluous.

As illustrated by the oversimplified example of a patient in diabetic coma, and as demonstrated more fully by the patient management problems included in the sample examination in Appendix B, this programmed testing technique may be likened to the linear method of programmed teaching rather than to the branching program method. Although the branching program method may seem attractive, and has been introduced by McGuire[7] as a modification of the PMP test, the National Board has held to the linear method to assure that each examinee is tested with essentially the same examination. When unlimited branching is permitted, two different examinees may take totally different approaches to the clinical situation and follow different pathways to the solution of the problem. In this case there is no accurate way to evaluate the two examinees except in terms of whether or not they ultimately solved the problem (e.g., gave the "correct" final diagnosis) regardless of what they had done (or not done) for the patient in the interim.

Failure on Part III

Who are the failures in Part III? Why should individuals fail, having acquired an M.D. degree in an approved medical school in the United States or Canada? Why should such individuals fail after having passed the Board's comprehensive examination in the clinical subjects (Part II) and in the basic medical sciences (Part I)?

In an attempt to answer these questions, scores of 145 candidates who failed a PMP examination were studied to determine the types of errors made. As

* The reliability of the total, full-day Part III examination, consisting of clinical material presented in graphic and pictorial form as well as the PMP section, is approximately .90.

pointed out earlier, in this examination it is possible to make two kinds of errors: errors of commission (choosing courses of action harmful to the patient) and errors of omission (failing to choose the courses of action beneficial to the patient). Theoretically, the poorest possible score on this test could be obtained by committing both of these types of errors, i.e., ordering all of the contraindicated measures and failing to order anything of benefit to the patient. However, none of the 145 candidates who failed the test behaved in this manner. Rather, the failures fell at either end of another dimension, apparently related to the number of decisions made. One type of failure is the "shotgunner" who orders a large number of studies or procedures. He commits relatively few errors of omission but, at the same time, he orders so many contraindicated procedures that even the most hardy patient would have difficulty in surviving. The other type of failure is the timid soul who makes very few choices lest he make a mistake. This candidate rarely makes an error of commission; his failure is in omitting procedures beneficial for his patient, and possibly even lifesaving.

These two types of young physician, the "shotgunner" and the timid soul, were quite clearly identified by the critical incident study forming the basis for the development of the PMP test. As noted in that study, the most frequently recorded examples of poor or inappropriate clinical practice observed among interns included: making a diagnosis with inadequate information (the timid soul) and prescribing medication with inadequate indication (the shotgunner). It is these physicians who, as failures on Part III, are judged by the National Board as not yet ready to be licensed for the practice of medicine, with full responsibility for the care and well-being of patients.

References

1. Hubbard, J. P.: Programmed testing in medicine. In *Testing Problems in Perspective* (Anastasi, A., Ed.). American Council of Education, Washington, 1966.
2. Hubbard, J. P., Levit, E. J., Schumacher, C. F. and Schnabel, T. C.: An objective evaluation of clinical competence. N. Engl. J. Med., 272:1321, 1965.
3. Fitzpatrick, R., et al.: *Development of Objective Flight Checks and Proficiency Measures for Use with Bombers, Reconnaissance and Cargo Crews*. American Institute of Research, Pittsburgh, 1954.
4. Flanagan, J. C.: The critical requirements approach to educational objectives. School and Society, 71:321, 1950.
5. Gordon, T.: The development of a standard flight check for the airline transport rating based on the critical requirements of the airline pilot's job. Report 85, Civil Aeronautics Administration, Washington, 1949.
6. Rimoldi, H. J. A.: Rationale and application of tests of diagnostic skill. J. Med. Educ., 38:364, 1963.
7. McGuire, C.: A process approach to the construction and analysis of medical examinations. J. Med. Educ., 38:556, 1963.

CHAPTER 5

■

Scoring and Analysis

Charles F. Schumacher

This chapter describes the scoring procedures and psychometric analyses applied to National Board examinations after they have been administered to large groups of examinees. No attempt is made to describe or even enumerate all techniques of scoring and analysis; these may be found in many excellent texts on psychometric methodology.[1-7] The methods currently being used by the National Board will be described in the light of twenty-five years of experience and continuous study. The concepts of scoring, item analysis and score conversion will be reviewed as they pertain to the series of National Board examinations, rather than as abstract psychometric principles.

This chapter will also consider the problem of ensuring the integrity of scores from certifying examinations—a problem in which a variety of information is examined and a decision is made regarding the "validity" of the scores obtained by an individual candidate. Much of the information involved may be provided by psychometric analysis of an examination or the examination performance of individual examinees, and thus the topic is included in this chapter. The reader should recognize, however, that this process is basically a judgmental one which goes far beyond the traditional realm of psychometrics.

Scoring

As pointed out earlier, the rightness or wrongness of each response to multiple-choice questions is predetermined by the panel of subject-matter specialists who write the questions and approve them for inclusion in the examination. The examinee makes his choice of the correct response as he takes the examination and records this choice on a special answer sheet. The first step in scoring is then to count the correct responses. Various scoring machines are used, depending in part upon the number of answer sheets to be scored and the urgency with which results must be reported. If very few individuals, or possibly a single individual, are to be examined, machine scoring may not be justified and the scoring may then be done by hand. Template forms are available or may be designed to provide for holes to be punched over the location of the correct response on the answer sheet. It is then an easy matter to count the correct responses appearing through the holes.

For the scoring of any multiple-choice test, a decision must be made as to which scoring formula will be used. When the examination is one in which all, or nearly all, examinees are given enough time to consider every item and are encouraged to record an answer for each item based upon whatever information they may have, the problem of selecting a scoring formula is largely academic. In this situation, scores based upon the number of questions answered correctly will rank examinees in the same way as scores based upon a formula in which a penalty is imposed for each wrong answer.[5] Moreover, scoring formulae that penalize examinees for "guessing" assume that all examinees take the same attitude toward a question for which they are not absolutely sure of the correct answer. Such an assumption ignores individual differences among examinees with respect to the personality characteristics influencing risk-taking. A calculated risk by one student may well be considered a wild guess by another. In National Board examinations, examinees are encouraged to answer all questions; no penalty is imposed for wrong answers. The scoring is then based only on the number of questions answered correctly.

A second important issue related to scoring is the question of whether or not to assign differential weights to different test items or to the various alternative answers for individual items. Differential weighting has been a topic of perennial debate in the psychological and educational literature, with conflicting results regarding the utility of this process for increasing the reliability or validity of an examination. In-house studies conducted by the National Board have suggested that Board examinations, as currently constructed, yield essentially the same results when items are weighted equally as they do when differential weights are applied. Therefore, currently, differential weighting is not used in scoring. However, studies of the effects of differential weighting of the various possible answers to individual items and additional studies of the effects of applying different weights at the item level are being conducted as part of the ongoing program of research and development at the National Board. These studies will undoubtedly have an effect upon the weighting strategy to be used in future Board examinations.

Item Analysis

It is axiomatic that the quality of an examination can be no better than the quality of the individual items which make up that examination. To monitor and improve an examination instrument, therefore, it is essential to develop methods for analyzing the performance of the individual items in that instrument. Perhaps the most important factor in judging the quality of a test item is the relevance of that item to the particular measurement purpose to be served by the examination. One must be concerned with the *validity* of the item for assessing some small segment of knowledge, facet of problem solving, aspect of judgment or limited skill which, when combined with additional similar measures, will provide a useful overall measurement of some competency that is important to the performance of a task such as the practice of medicine.

Validation of individual test items is no easy task and yet it is probably the most important single step that can be taken to develop high-quality examinations.

Procedures employed by the National Board to validate its test items include ongoing review by the test committees and periodic external studies of the relevance of test items.

The relevance of test items to the objectives of medical education is a factor that does not lend itself to expression in numerical values. It is a judgmental concept related to what the examiner thinks the examinee should know and is subject to interpretations of the aims of medical education and of the degree to which a particular question or problem may be directly related to such aims. The range of such interpretations is wide and growing wider as the educational system endeavors to adjust to the massive quantity of medical knowledge and to decide what, from this overwhelming mass, should be included in the medical school curriculum.

The resulting uncertainties and changing curricular patterns create a formidable challenge for the examination system. The National Board's answer to this challenge lies in the collective judgment of its corps of examiners—about 110 representatives of the educational system. However, even the judgment of 110 distinguished medical educators currently active in the educational process on a national basis may be questioned by an individual medical school.

Repetitive studies have been undertaken by the National Board to determine the degree to which the grades resulting from its examinations do in fact agree with the independent judgment of medical school faculties in ranking their own students. At the very outset of the National Board's use of multiple-choice tests during the academic year 1952-53, medical schools in which all or nearly all students were then taking National Board examinations were asked to provide, prior to the examinations, ratings of the proficiency of students in the subjects of the tests. These ratings were simply listings of students designating the top fifth, middle three-fifths and lower fifth of the class in each subject. As reported by Cowles and Hubbard,[8] correlations of test scores and faculty ratings were very satisfactory, demonstrating that the results of these early National Board examinations did correspond closely with the appraisal of students by their own faculties. Similar studies, carried out subsequently with larger numbers of participating medical school classes, have yielded similar results.

During the academic years 1969-70 and 1970-71, a different approach to determining the judgment of the medical educational community about the validity and relevance of National Board examinations was undertaken.* The Board committed itself to a rather bold and forthright undertaking: to ask and to answer, for all to see, how National Board examinations fit the educational objectives of medical schools. A further question could have been asked: whether the educational objectives are adequately oriented to the needs of society. Exploration of this latter question, however, was not viewed as the task of the National Board. The Board's function remains that of measuring fully and fairly what is being taught in medical school today, leaving to others the determination of what ought to be taught.

The data resulting from this study were, on the whole, reassuring: 90 per cent of the questions in the basic medical sciences were judged by two-thirds or more of the basic-science departments to represent important knowledge

* The National Board of Medical Examiners is indebted to the Carnegie Corporation and The Commonwealth Fund for financial support for this research study.

relevant to their disciplines. The view of clinical faculties when they too judged basic-science questions was expectedly variable. Nevertheless, 83 per cent of the questions in basic medical science were considered relevant by one or more of the clinical departments. A similar assessment of clinical-science questions by clinical departments also gave a reassuring view of the relevance of individual clinical-science questions.

Given that an examination question is judged to be relevant to the purpose of the examination, it may still fail to contribute to the overall mission of the examination if it is not at an appropriate level of difficulty for the particular population of examinees to whom the test will be administered or if it fails to measure that area of knowledge or kind of competency that is measured by the test as a whole. Fortunately, there are numerical indices for judging these aspects of item performance. These are calculated routinely for all items that appear in National Board examinations.

Item Difficulty (P value)

The difficulty of an individual item is generally defined* as the percentage (P) of some specified group of examinees that answer the item correctly. The higher this percentage, the easier the item. A P value of .95 would indicate that 95 per cent of the examinees responded to the item correctly and that this particular item presented very little difficulty to the examinees; nearly all knew the right answer. An item with such a high P value contributes virtually nothing to the test. It does no harm; neither does it do any good. It has the effect of giving an extra point to the examinees, good and poor alike. If, on the other hand, the P value is very low, either the item may be too difficult for the group being tested or the item itself may be defective. A choice considered wrong by the committee of examiners (a distracter) may, for one reason or another, be considered correct by a large proportion of the examinees. A P value approaching .20 for a five-choice item or .25 for a four-choice item suggests that the examinees may be indulging in chance guessing without real knowledge of the particular point or question. In such cases, the test item is carefully considered together with its index of discrimination (r_{bis}, described below) and a decision made as to whether it should be deleted from the examination in the final scoring procedure (see pages 53, 54).

In the experience of the National Board, there is a wide range of difficulty in the test items first introduced into an examination, although the average P value is usually between .60 and .65. When the examiners review the performance of candidates on individual items, they find many surprises. How could 40 per cent of medical students or residents not have known the answer to a question that the examiners had thought all should know? Sometimes an examiner goes so far as to say: "If a student does not know the answer to that question he should not pass the test!" Such an item is tagged, and the P value is brought to the attention of the examiners the following year. Examiners may then learn the fallibility of judging students on the basis of their own feelings for a single question.

---

* Item difficulty has a different meaning in the context of a relatively new theory of measurement known as "latent-trait" theory. For an introduction to this particular area of psychometrics the reader is referred to the *Journal of Educational Measurement*, 14:73, 1977.

Item Discrimination (r$_{bis}$)

A second numerical index of the quality of an individual test item is the correlation coefficient between the item and the total test (or major segment of the total test) in which the item appeared. This statistic provides a measure of the extent to which a single item measures the general area of knowledge, skill or ability that is being measured by the test as a whole (or the major section of the test). If the test measures an important competency, individual items should also measure that same competency to be included in the overall score derived from the test. The item-discrimination index (also known as the item-test correlation) allows one to judge the extent to which an individual item can distinguish (discriminate) between examinees who score well on the total test and those who score poorly.

A number of indices of discrimination have been developed over the years to fit a variety of testing situations. The index used by the National Board is the biserial correlation coefficient (r$_{bis}$). This particular index has certain advantages over other possible indices when the data to which it is applied meet the assumptions underlying its use. Generally, it is most appropriate when examinee groups are large and when the characteristic being measured by both the items and the total test is continuous and approximately normally distributed. These assumptions appear to be met quite well by our data.

A biserial correlation coefficient may be calculated directly or it may be approximated reasonably accurately from published tables.[9] Until recently, the labor involved in calculating this index directly for a large number of items (roughly 1000 in Part I or Part II) has been almost prohibitive, and approximate methods are accurate enough for most practical purposes. Now the advent of high-speed, large-capacity computers has made it unnecessary to settle for approximations (even very good ones) and the direct method of calculation is used almost universally.

The formula for the direct calculation of this index is:

$$r_{bis} = \left(\frac{M_p - M_t}{S_t}\right) \ \left(\frac{P}{y}\right)$$

where r$_{bis}$ = biserial correlation between an item score and the subtest score to which the item belongs

M$_p$ = mean subtest score for those examinees who answered the item correctly

M$_t$ = mean subtest score for all examinees

S$_t$ = raw score standard deviation for the total group on the subtest

P = proportion of the group that answered the item correctly

y = ordinate of the unit-normal distribution at point P (the point *above* which P proportion of the area under that curve will fall)

To obtain a better "feel" for the information provided by this index, it is also helpful to understand a widely used procedure for approximating the biserial correlation coefficient. This procedure employs data from two groups of examinees whose performances on the total test are either very good or very poor. Scores are obtained for a sample of examinees and a frequency distribution of these scores is obtained. The two groups employed in the calculation of item discrimination indices consist of those examinees in the upper 27 per cent (high group) and in the lower 27 per cent (low group) of this distribution. For each item in the test, the percentage of examinees in each of these two groups that answered that item correctly is calculated. These percentages (labeled P High and P Low respectively) are then used as arguments for entering a published table from which the approximate value of r_{bis} for the item is obtained. In using this approach, one quickly learns that the magnitude of the biserial correlation increases as the *difference* between P High and P Low increases. In the extreme, when P High = 100 (the item is answered correctly by all members of the high group) and P Low = 0 (no one in the low group answered the item correctly), the value of r_{bis} = 1.0 (its maximum positive value). Such an item "discriminates" perfectly between those who have a high degree of the knowledge, skill or ability that is measured by the total test and those who have relatively little of this knowledge, skill or ability. If P High and P Low are equal (no matter what their magnitude) r_{bis} will be zero, indicating that the item *cannot* distinguish between the more-knowledgeable and the less-knowledgeable groups. Finally, if P Low is greater than P High, the discrimination index for the item will be negative in sign, suggesting that the particular item in question is measuring something that is *inversely* related to the knowledge or other characteristic that is being measured by the total test. When an item in a National Board examination has a negative discrimination index which is of sufficient magnitude to rule out simply a chance occurrence (generally −.25 or higher in the negative direction), it is reviewed very carefully for possible ambiguities or other flaws which might account for such performance so that corrective action, if indicated, can be taken before the item is used in a subsequent examination or, under certain circumstances, to exclude the item from the final scoring of an examination as described below under *Key Validation*.

From the foregoing, it should be clear that the item discrimination index provides a measure of the extent to which an item "fits" with the total test. Tests which are composed of items having high discrimination indices are characterized as "homogeneous" or "unidimensional," since they tend to measure a single area or domain rather than a conglomerate of several different unrelated areas of knowledge, abilities or skills. Indirectly, a high degree of homogeneity supports the content validity of the examination since it suggests that the test author has defined a domain of knowledge or an ability that is more than simply a collection of unrelated units. High overall discrimination also indicates that items appear to come from this common domain and "hang together" to form a meaningful total picture, rather than standing as a collection of unrelated bits of information.

Key Validation

National Board examinations are newly created each year to assure that they are current and in step with the rapid advances in medical knowledge. New test items are, however, subject to the hazards of newness. Despite the wise judgment and agreement of panels of experts, the difficulty (P value) or index of discrimination (r_{bis}) of individual items cannot be predicted accurately. A new question may be too difficult or too easy for the examinee population; it may have more than one correct answer that has escaped the closest attention of the examiners; it may contain undetected ambiguities or other technical flaws. Even though the question has been constructed with care, edited diligently and reviewed by several subject-matter experts, the real test of the question is the test of use.

For many practical reasons, among which is the necessity of maintaining the security of the Board's examinations, it has not been considered practical or advisable to pretest items on a selected group of students before an examination is given for purposes of qualification and certification. Until recently, therefore, it has been impossible to keep an examination current by including large numbers of new questions and, at the same time, to pretest the new questions for clarity, appropriateness, difficulty level, discrimination and freedom from technical error.

With the advent of high-speed scoring equipment and computer hardware, it is now possible to obtain an accurate estimate of the performance of each individual test question after the examination has been administered but before final scores are obtained. The process by which this is accomplished has been labeled "key validation." After an examination has been administered, a random sample of examinees is chosen, their answer sheets are scored according to the answer key established by the test committee and a full item analysis (see page 49) is performed on the examination. Individual test questions that perform poorly in terms of difficulty and discrimination are identified and reviewed in detail by a psychometric staff member and a medical staff member. On the basis of their review and after consultation with the committee responsible for the test, individual questions performing poorly can be deleted from the examination when the final scoring of the test is done. Thus, it is possible to test each item against the criterion of performance before allowing it to influence the score of any examinee.

Score Conversion

In an ongoing examination program in which a number of subscores are extracted from each form of the test, it is necessary to provide some mechanism by which scores may be compared from year to year in a particular subject, and from subject to subject within a particular examination. Because examinations may differ in length, item difficulty and item discrimination, raw scores (number of questions answered correctly) will almost certainly not be comparable from year to year or from subject to subject. Several different approaches are available to convert raw scores to some other scale which will permit comparisons. A simple example is the conversion of raw scores to percentage scores. This operation makes it possible to compare tests of different lengths if it can be assumed that the tests are similar with respect to other characteristics, such as item difficulty. Unfortunately, however, examinations differ in more ways than simply the number of questions they contain; thus merely converting raw scores to percentage scores is rarely satisfactory.

The conversion system used by the National Board and by many other testing agencies is a linear conversion system; the converted score is derived by applying two constants to the raw score. In its most general form, this system can be expressed by the following equation:

$$Y = a + bX \qquad \text{(Eq. 1)}$$

where Y is the converted score
        X is the raw score
        a and b are empirically determined constants

From this equation it is apparent that converted scores can differ widely from each other, depending upon the constants chosen. In fact, the final scale on which converted scores are expressed depends completely upon the manner in which these constants are derived.

One method of determining constants results in what has been labeled "standard scores." Standard scores are used for National Board examinations, for specialty board examinations, aptitude testing and achievement testing programs in many fields. In addition to correcting for differences in test length, standard scores provide a means for correcting for differences in test difficulty and in discrimination level, reflected in the raw score means and raw score standard deviations respectively.

Standard scores are defined as follows:

$$Z = \frac{X - \overline{X}}{SD_x} \qquad \text{(Eq. 2)}$$

where Z = standard score
      X = raw score
      $\overline{X}$ = mean raw score of a reference group
   SD_x = raw score standard deviation of the
           reference group

When this basic equation is used, standard scores of the reference group will have a mean of zero, a standard deviation of 1, and, if the distribution of scores is symmetric, half of the standard scores will be negative in sign. In many instances it is more convenient to work with scores with a higher mean (e.g., 500), a larger standard deviation (e.g., 100), and positive signs. The requirements can be met by simply adding appropriate constants to Equation 2 as follows:

$$Z = 100 \left[\frac{X - \overline{X}}{SD_x} \right] + 500 \qquad \text{(Eq. 3)}$$

Standard scores calculated according to Equation 3 will have a mean of 500 and a standard deviation of 100, regardless of the mean and standard deviation of the raw scores from which they were derived, and will rank examinees in exactly the same way as standard scores obtained using Equation 2.

The equation for converting raw scores to standard scores (Equation 2) may also be expressed as:

(Eq. 4)

$$Z = \left(\frac{-\overline{X}}{SD_x}\right) + \left[\frac{1}{SD_x}(X)\right]$$

Equation 4 then is Equation 1 in which the a constant is defined as $\frac{-\overline{X}}{SD_x}$ and the b constant as $\frac{1}{SD_x}$. Thus, the equation for converting raw scores to standard scores is a linear conversion equation. Because linear conversions do not alter the order of individual scores, examinees will be ranked in the same way on the basis of their standard scores as they are on the basis of their original raw scores.

A somewhat different linear conversion was used until recently for National Board examinations in order to be able to report passing scores as 75 or higher. Since this had been traditional in days of essay tests, medical schools and students were familiar with this passing level and many state boards of medical licensure had it written into state law. Also from the essay tests, 88 or above was recognized as an honor score. These two points, 75 as the passing level and 88 as the honor level, were two key scores that established the scale upon which this conversion was based. These two scores therefore had the same meaning over time and from test to test. The linear equation from converting raw scores to these "scale scores" (not to be confused with the standard scores described above) was derived by solving the following set of simultaneous equations:

$$U(a) + b = 88 \qquad \text{(Eq. 5)}$$
$$L(a) + b = 75 \qquad \text{(Eq. 6)}$$

where U = the raw score defining "honor"
performance
L = the raw score defining minimum
passing performance

Subtracting Equation 6 from Equation 5 yields an equation in one unknown (a) which can be solved. Once the value of a has been determined, this value can be inserted into either Equation 5 or Equation 6 to find the required value of b which will satisfy both equations. The a and b constants derived in this manner are then inserted into Equation 1 and used to convert all raw scores to scale scores. Again, because scale scores are derived from a linear conversion equation, examinees would be ranked in the same order by their scale scores as by their original raw scores.

From the foregoing discussion it is apparent that the conversion process is necessary in the handling of score information to provide the test user with data comparable from test to test and from year to year. It should also be apparent that the conversion process has no necessary relationship to the setting of standards for passing or failing an examination. Standard setting (see pages 67 to 71) is a judgmental process by which a certifying agency defines the lowest level of performance on an examination acceptable for purposes of certification. Score conversion, on the other hand, is a mechanical operation which may be performed on any set of scores, regardless of whether or not a standard is established for the test from which these scores are obtained.

Integrity of National Board Credentials

Scores and certificates such as those issued by the National Board are credentials. They are concise and precise means by which individuals may convey to others information concerning the extent and quality of certain of their achievements. Obviously, the achievements implied by certification of the National Board are in the realm of problem solving, clinical management and the acquisition of medical knowledge, both scientific and clinical.

For several years the value to individuals of their National Board credentials has been increasing. Certification after successful completion of all three parts of the Board examinations is recognized for purposes of medical licensure by nearly all jurisdictions. Additionally, the schedule for acquiring this certification is convenient for medical students, who can acquire Part I and Part II during the course of their medical studies and often in conjunction with the examination programs of their schools. This latter feature, however, emphasizes another value placed on National Board scores, because some schools use them as important elements in evaluating students for promotion. There are also increasing reports of requests by residency program directors for Part I and Part II scores to be used in the process of selecting applicants who have attended schools without a grading scale.

For another group of students, a partial National Board examination record has acquired a value that was never anticipated when the examination was first designed. Students in foreign medical schools, especially American citizens, now use Part 1 scores as an essential credential in support of their applications for transfer to advanced standing in American medical schools. The National Board has cooperated with the Association of American Medical Colleges in the Coordinated Transfer Application System (COTRANS) and with individual schools in programs for the evaluation of students whose applications are under consideration by the school. Applicants involved in these transfer processes naturally tend to look upon their scores as being vitally important to their personal futures.

Involvement with students or graduates of foreign medical schools has become more intense and more complicated as a result of the National Board examinations having been specifically mentioned in the recently enacted federal Health Professions Educational Assistance Act of 1976 as required for all alien foreign medical graduates who apply for immigration to the United States. This requirement led to the development of the Visa Qualifying Examination (VQE) as described in Chapter 8.

These conditions offer immediate rewards for successful scores and undoubtedly supply a temptation to seek every possible advantage in preparing for and taking the examinations.

The value of credentials such as National Board scores or certification depends upon their having a recognized validity, which in turn has two important components: (1) The evaluations must be properly related to the achievements they aim to measure and (2) the measurements must be made under conditions which are standard for all examinees and harmonious with the design of the evaluation procedure. While concerns for validity generally focus on the first of these two components, the second is also of critical importance and cannot be taken for granted. A critical question is: Have all examinees completed the examination in compliance with the conditions and rules which it was assumed that they would follow during the entire evaluation process?

As noted in Chapter 2, selected, previously used test items are included in well-designed examinations to increase the efficiency and reliability of the evaluation and to provide a means of assuring equivalence among scores on various administrations of different versions of the examination. To accomplish this purpose, the National Board places the greatest importance on maintaining the security of its examinations and all individual questions, for all of which the Board holds the copyright. (The *only* questions that have ever been released from this security since the introduction of multiple-choice questions are those included in the appendix of this volume and its first edition.)

The ready availability of copying devices has, however, placed unaccustomed strains upon this prime requisite of the Board's examinations. It has therefore become essential to tighten the procedures for the security of the examinations before, during and following their administration and also to introduce new, sophisticated, carefully studied checks in the scoring of the answer papers.

In other professions and occupations, credentials often confer benefits principally upon their owner, but those of physicians give them the privilege of the practice of medicine, with its grave attendant responsibilities. The integrity of such credentials is of important concern to many, other than the physicians themselves, and each instance of invalid credentials is potentially damaging to patients, the public and other candidates who hold National Board certification. Therefore, the National Board places the highest priority on efforts to protect the integrity of the credentials it grants to examinees.

References

1. Anastasi, A.: *Psychological Testing*, 3rd ed. The Macmillan Company, New York, 1968.
2. Ebel, R. L.: *Essentials of Educational Measurement*. Prentice-Hall, Englewood Cliffs, 1972.
3. Guilford, J. P.: *Fundamental Statistics in Psychology and Education*, 3rd ed. McGraw-Hill, New York, 1956.
4. Gulliksen, H.: *Theory of Mental Tests*. John Wiley and Sons, New York, 1950.
5. Hubbard, J. P. and Clemans, W. Y.: *Multiple-choice Examinations in Medicine*. Lea & Febiger, Philadelphia, 1961.
6. Lindquist, E. F. (Ed.): *Educational Measurement*. American Council on Education, Washington, 1951.
7. Thorndike, R. L. (Ed.): *Educational Measurement*. American Council on Education, Washington, 1971.
8. Cowles, J. T. and Hubbard, J. P.: Validity and reliability of the new objective tests. J. Med. Educ., 29(6):30, 1954.
9. Fan, Chung-teh: *Item Analysis Table*. Educational Testing Service, Princeton, 1952.

CHAPTER 6

■

Reliability, Validity and Standard Setting

Charles F. Schumacher

Examinations, viewed as instruments for the measurement of medical knowledge or skill, must have the same characteristics expected of other dependable instruments. They must yield consistent results that can be relied upon from one administration to the next; they must be designed to test what they are intended to test; they must have the capacity to distinguish between individuals who have met some standard of excellence and those who have not. These three properties are described as follows under the headings of reliability, validity and standard setting.

Reliability

Reliability has been defined in a number of ways, but the most useful definition appears to be one that considers reliability as the capacity of an instrument to provide measures reproducible over time. Instruments used for measuring common physical properties (rulers, scales, thermometers) generally have a high degree of reliability in this sense, so high, in fact, that users of such instruments rarely need to be concerned about this important property of measuring instruments in general. Examinations are a very different kind of instrument and the measurements made by them, i.e., examination scores, are subject to all of the complex factors that produce variability in human behavior. Therefore, tests are not as likely to provide reliable (reproducible) measurements as are instruments that measure simple physical characteristics. Some of the factors influencing behavior (such as learning) are precisely the ones an examination attempts to measure; others (such as the emotional state of the examinee during the test) may produce unwanted variability in examination scores and thus reduce the degree to which the test will yield consistent results. The question of reliability, therefore, assumes major importance in evaluating any testing procedure.

A high degree of reliability alone does not guarantee that an examination will measure that which it is designed to measure. For example, a highly reliable test of medical knowledge might not be appropriate for measuring a physician's attitude toward patients. However, an examination that appears to measure important characteristics but has low reliability may be worse than no examination at all. Such instruments will almost certainly provide misinformation about the characteristics of individual examinees, and may lead to erroneous conclusions about the value of various educational programs if the test performance of groups of examinees is used as a criterion for judging these programs.

Ideally, the reliability of an examination would be measured by administering the test at least twice to a representative group of the examinees for whom the examination was designed and then calculating the correlation coefficient between the scores obtained on the two administrations of the test. However, in addition to the practical problems involved, this approach encounters the potentially serious problem of "practice effect" from the first administration of the test. Individuals may remember test questions from one administration to another and, therefore, the examinee group may be expected to change as a result of the first administration. Their performance on the second administration, then, is a function both of the reliability of the test and of the effect of having taken the test once before, and the correlation between their scores on the two testings will probably not provide an accurate estimate of the reliability of the instrument.

An alternative approach to estimating test reliability requires only one administration of the test. In this procedure (split-half technique), the examination is divided into two half tests (e.g. odd-numbered questions assigned to one half and even-numbered questions assigned to the other half); scores are then obtained for each half test and the correlation coefficient between the half tests is calculated.

It has been demonstrated[1] that one of the characteristics of a test having a direct influence upon its reliability is its length. Thus, the final step in calculating reliability with the split-half technique is to estimate the size of the correlation coefficient between the half-test scores (reliability coefficient) for a test twice as long as either of the halves, i.e., for the test as a whole. This is done by applying the following formula (a version of the Spearman-Brown prophecy formula) to the correlation coefficient between the half tests:

$$r_T = \frac{2r_H}{1 + r_H}$$

where r_T = the reliability coefficient
for the test as a whole

r_H = the correlation coefficient
between the half tests

The split-half method of estimating reliability eliminates the problem of "practice effect." This approach is not entirely satisfactory, however, because there are many ways in which a test may be divided into two halves.* Any

* If there are 2N items in a test there are $\frac{(2N)!}{2(N)!(N)!}$ ways in which these items may be divided into half tests each of which contains N items. For example, there are 92,378 ways in which a test of 20 items could be split into two half tests of 10 items each.

method chosen for splitting the test will be somewhat arbitrary, and the resulting reliability coefficient will be slightly different from the one that would have been obtained if a different method of splitting the test had been used.

The dilemma can be resolved when individual item statistics are available for an examination. The reliability of the test can then be estimated so that only one solution is provided and all of the possible interactions between examinees and individual items are taken into consideration. In a sense this technique treats each individual question as a subtest, rather than concentrating on only two of the many half tests that could be considered. A number of investigators [2-4] have explored this general approach to estimating test reliability and in 1937 Kuder and Richardson[5] published a series of formulae for calculating test reliability from individual item statistics. One of these formulae has been widely accepted by psychometricians as a substantial improvement over the split-half technique. Known as Kuder-Richardson Formula 20, it is currently used for estimating the reliability of many examinations, including most of the tests prepared by the National Board. It is as follows:

$$r = \frac{K}{K-1} \left[\frac{S^2 - \sum\limits_{i=1}^{K} p_i \, q_i}{S^2} \right]$$

where r = the reliability coefficient for
the examination

K = the number of scorable units (items)
in the examination

S = the standard deviation of the test
in raw-score units

p_i = the percentage of examinees answering
the ith question correctly (the P value
for the ith question)

$q_i = 1 - p_i$

Even though the Kuder-Richardson technique differs from the split-half method with respect to the way in which the reliability coefficient is calculated, the K-R 20 coefficient may be considered as a generalized form of split-half reliability such as one might obtain by averaging all of the split-half coefficients that would be obtained if an examination were in fact divided into all possible pairs of half tests and a correlation coefficient calculated for each pair.

Another valuable investigation of the properties of the K-R 20 coefficient was done by Swineford[6] in 1959. She showed that the K-R 20 reliability coefficient can be estimated fairly accurately simply from the number of items in the test and the mean discrimination index (r_{bis}) of those items. Thus, the two major factors determining the reliability of a test are test length (as indicated earlier) and the "quality" of individual test questions in terms of their ability to discriminate between criterion groups of examinees.

All of the indices of reliability cited above are expressed as correlation coefficients with maximum values of 1.00. In interpreting the reliability coefficient, the question arising immediately is a practical one: How large must this correlation coefficient be in order that the test user may have confidence in the testing instrument? While no precise answer can be given, the following guidelines used by the National Board may be helpful:

1. If the reliability coefficient for an examination is less than .70, scores from that test should not be used for evaluation of individuals or groups.
2. If an examination is to be used only for comparing the performance of groups of individuals (e.g., mean scores of school classes or groups of physicians) a reliability coefficient of .70 or higher is acceptable.
3. If an examination is to be used to distinguish between individual examinees (e.g., candidates for certification), the reliability coefficient should be .90 or higher.

The reliability coefficient for a test is directly related to another statistical property of the examination also of value in judging the accuracy with which the test measures. This statistic is known as the standard error of measurement and is defined as follows:

$$\text{SEM} = S\sqrt{1 - r}$$

where SEM = the standard error of measurement

S = the standard deviation of test scores

r = the reliability coefficient for the test

The standard error of measurement provides a means of determining the range within which the scores of an individual examinee might be expected to vary by chance alone at a specified level of probability if he were tested again with the same examination and if no "practice effect" had occurred as a result of the first test with the same examination.* It should be noted that the size of the SEM (and, therefore, the range within which a score might vary by chance alone) decreases in relation to the square root of the reliability coefficient. Thus, a test with a reliability of .75 yields a SEM of about one-half of a standard deviation unit, whereas a reliability of .90 reduces the SEM to only about one-third of a standard deviation and a reliability of .95 shrinks the SEM still further to less than one-fourth of a standard deviation.

---

* Assuming that an examination with a reliability coefficient of .95 yielded scores having a standard deviation of 5 points, the SEM would be 1.1. The chances are about 2 to 1 that an examinee who obtained a score of 80 on this test would obtain a score between 79 and 81 if he were tested again with the same test.

The important aspects of reliability as it pertains to achievement testing may be summarized as follows:

1. A high degree of reliability is a necessary but not sufficient condition for a good examination.
2. The reliability of a test can be estimated accurately from information obtained from a single administration of the test.
3. Reliability is a function of *test length* (number of items) and *quality* (discriminating power) of the individual items within the test.
4. If an examination is to be used for distinguishing between *individual examinees*, a higher degree of reliability is necessary than if the test is to be used only for comparing the performances of *groups*.
5. The precision with which a test measures increases as the square root of the reliability coefficient. Thus, fairly small increments in the reliability coefficient can produce rather large improvements in precision.

Validity

Perhaps *the* most important question that can be asked about any measuring instrument is: To what extent does the instrument measure those characteristics of examinees that it is intended to measure? A synonymous question would be: How valid is the instrument? Thus, the concept of test validity is concerned with *what* the examination measures and the *degree to which* a test, or other measuring instrument, measures certain characteristics that the test author and test user are interested in measuring.

A test is not "valid" or "invalid," rather, it has some degree of validity for some particular purpose. Also, most tests have some degree of validity for measuring certain characteristics of examinees but rarely, if ever, would a test be able to measure *all* of the characteristics that would be required for the examinee to perform a complex series of behaviors such as those behaviors that must be performed by the "competent physician." The important attributes of this concept are that validity is concerned with *what* is being measured and the *extent to which* it is being measured by a particular instrument.

There are several ways in which the test constructor may seek to answer the question concerning the validity of a given instrument. Each of these validation strategies provides a different approach to the definition of what is being measured and, consequently, we can refer to several different *types* of validity depending upon the particular strategy that has been used for a given examination. Three major generic types of validity have been defined and are now generally accepted by the measurement community: content validity, construct validity and criterion-related validity. Excellent technical definitions for these may be found in "Standards for Educational and Psychological Tests," which was prepared in 1974 by a joint committee of the APA, AERA and NCME. In our discussion, we will attempt to translate them into the context of examinations designed to test medical students and physicians, recognizing that we may lose some precision in the process. As we describe each major type of validity, we will also discuss the efforts that have been made (and those which are currently being made) to establish a particular type of validity or to estimate the degree to which it is present in National Board examinations.

Content Validity

Validation efforts that focus on the content validity of a test consider that which is to be measured as some well-defined area of knowledge, ability or skill, often referred to as a *domain*. A precise definition of the domain is an essential step in the validation efforts. One critical element in the establishment of content validity is evidence that the test constructor has developed a clear, detailed, logical description of the particular domain which the test will be built to measure.

Most domains of interest in medical certifying examinations are large enough so that one could never feasibly test for all of the knowledge, abilities or skills that constitute the entire domain. Therefore, it is essential that a rational method be established for sampling from the domain to produce a testing instrument that is representative of the entire domain. Content-validation studies, therefore, are also very much concerned with the sampling methods used to construct the examination and the extent to which the test matches with the description of the domain that preceded test construction.

This type of validation (unlike the other types) does not yield a numeric index of the degree of validity that a given instrument may have. Rather, it is a judgment based upon evidence that the test constructor has logically and clearly defined what is to be tested, developed test items which relate to this definition and constructed a testing instrument which faithfully represents those areas of knowledge or skill that appear in the original definition.

Because content validity is not quantifiable, it is sometimes confused with "face validity," which is the superficial impression that an instrument measures what it was intended to measure without any real definition of the domain or any deliberate effort to sample from it in a representative, rational manner. Face validity is rarely, if ever, acceptable as the only type of evidence that a test measures what it was intended to measure. Content validation, on the other hand, may be the most important type of validation strategy in an ongoing examination program in which new examination instruments are created fairly often and where it would be absolutely impractical to conduct other types of validation efforts for each new test. This is precisely the situation in which the National Board and most agencies that develop certifying examinations in medicine find themselves. Therefore, much of the validation efforts of these testing agencies is devoted to the establishment of the content validity of their examinations. Other types of validation are also done on a periodic basis, but each new test must possess a high degree of content validity in order to serve as a useful tool in the certification process. The process by which National Board examinations are designed and constructed is described in detail in Chapter 2, and therefore will not be repeated here. The reason for the painstaking process employed, however, should be clear from the foregoing discussion of content validity. Only by a process in which much time and effort of many knowledgeable examiners are devoted to the definition of what is to be tested and then to the development of specific test material to match these definitions is a testing agency able to give assurance to examinees and to the public that its tests possess a high degree of content validity.

Construct Validity

In establishing the construct validity of an examination, one seeks to explain differences in test scores on the basis of some underlying trait or characteristic of the examinee that can be measured by some means independent of the particular test in question. An example might be the "construct" of "clinical problem solving." We postulate that examinees differ with respect to the amount of "clinical problem solving" they possess and seek ways outside of the examination we have built to measure this underlying, nonobservable trait. One somewhat crude measure might be the level of medical training that groups have attained at the time they are tested. Our assumption in using this measure would be that individuals learn to solve clinical problems as they progress through clinical clerkships and begin to take an increasing amount of responsibility for the care of patients. Thus, examinees who are in an internship or residency training program should have more clinical-problem-solving ability than students who are just beginning their clinical clerkship experience. If we test both groups and find clearly superior performance by the intern-resident group, we would have at least preliminary evidence of the construct validity of our test. We would, of course, also want to exercise certain experimental or statistical controls to ensure that our results were not due to some extraneous factor(s) (difference in age, intellectual capacity, fund of medical information, etc.) and we might have difficulty in controlling all of these. However, if predictions about test performance made from several external measures of the "construct" match with actual performance of groups of examinees, additional evidence is accumulated to support the construct validity of the test.

A recent study of the construct validity of the National Board Part III followed essentially the strategy outlined above. In this study, the test performance of students at the end of the third year in medical school was compared with the performance of individuals near the end of their internship year on the same Part III examination. These groups were chosen on the assumption that interns, on the whole, should exhibit a greater degree of "clinical competence" than third-year students by virtue of the kinds of educational experience (increasing responsibility for patient care) normally occurring during the fourth year in medical school and during the internship. In terms of their Part III average score, 90 per cent of the third-year students fell below the mean of the intern group; differences of similar magnitude were found for each of the subsections of the Part III examination.[7]

An extension of this study, using the same basic procedure for identifying criterion groups, compared the performance of these same junior students with their subsequent performance on an equivalent Part III examination taken after they had completed eight months of their internship training. The results of this longitudinal study were almost identical with the results of the earlier cross-sectional study: The test performance at the internship level was again substantially better than performance as third-year students, with 91 per cent of the third-year scores falling below the mean internship score.

Criterion-related Validity

Studies of criterion-related validity define that which is to be measured as the behavior of the examinee in some task, which may range from actual on-the-job performance through performance in a simulated job situation to performance on another examination which itself has presumably been validated. Two subtypes of criterion-related validity are *concurrent* validity and *predictive* validity. The major difference between these subcategories is the relationship in time between the administration of the test and the collection of the criterion information. In studies of concurrent validity the test is administered and the criterion data are collected at approximately the same time, whereas in predictive validation studies criterion data are collected some time (months or even years) after the test has been administered. In either case, the validity of the test is generally estimated by calculating a correlation coefficient between test scores and criterion data.

An example of concurrent validity is to be found in the demonstration of correlations between National Board examination scores on the one hand and independent concurrent ratings of the same students provided by their medical schools on the other.[8-10] It was, in fact, the significance of these correlations in early studies undertaken jointly by the National Board and the Educational Testing Service (see Chapter 1) that, when added to the evidence of content validity alluded to above, led to the confidence in multiple-choice examinations and the discontinuation of the essay examination.

Predictive validity may appear to be the "best" or "most important" type of validity to establish for a certifying examination. However, real difficulties are inherent in conducting this type of validation study for examinations in medicine. As noted above, predictive validity deals with measurements at one point in the educational sequence in relation to criteria to be met by the same individuals at a later point in time. The ultimate in predictive validity for an examination in the broad field of medicine would be evidence that it predicts with a measurable degree of accuracy the "on-the-job" performance of the physician. However, there is no generally accepted method for measuring physician performance and, consequently, the criteria against which the earlier test scores may be matched are lacking. Moreover, studies of predictive validity require that a sample of examinees be tested and then, at some later date, these examinees be permitted to perform the "criterion" tasks that will be used to evaluate the testing instrument. Given that the social consequences of performing the criterion tasks badly are minimal, this strategy for validation is a sensible one. However, for the physician, the social consequences of performing badly are so great that this traditional model for investigating predictive validity would be unacceptable for medical certifying examinations. At best, studies of the predictive validity of such examinations are forced to employ samples of examinees in which the less-able individuals may be screened out between the time they take the test and the time at which criterion data are collected.

Do scores on National Board examinations predict success on specialty board examinations at a later point in the educational continuum? Such a question implies that performance on specialty board examinations might be substituted for measures of physician performance as the criterion measure in the predictive validity model. Indeed, it might even be argued that performance on specialty board examinations is an important criterion in its own right, since currently our society will permit only a relatively few physicians to pursue the particular type of medical career they have chosen unless they have been certified by some specialty board.

The National Board has investigated the correlation between performance on its Part II examination and later performance on the examinations of the three major specialty boards. These studies yielded a statistically significant positive correlation of moderate size in each instance. However, such validation efforts are not completely satisfying because the relationship between performance on specialty board examinations and eventual on-the-job performance is unknown.

Nevertheless, within limits, it is possible and fruitful to use the predictive validity model for certification examinations in medicine. In the development of a new examination for the purpose of determining whether a physician has acquired sufficient clinical competence for the supervised care of patients in a hospital setting, the National Board, at present writing, is undertaking a study of the results of an examination taken by fourth-year medical students to be compared with measurements of clinical competence of the same individuals at later dates in their training as residents. To the extent that these measurements of clinical competence are relevant and reliable indices of the on-the-job performance of residents, they should provide reasonable yardsticks against which the examination may be judged.

Establishing Grading Standards

The major purpose for creating any achievement test is to distinguish between individuals who have met some standard of excellence and those who have not. While testing instruments such as National Board examinations may also serve other useful purposes (e.g., providing diagnostic feedback to individual examinees, serving as a yardstick to help measure the effects of curricular change), the basic reason for these tests is to arrive at a decision as to whether an individual can be considered qualified for a license to practice medicine. Therefore, a crucial problem for the examination system is setting a standard for passing or failing the test.

In order to establish a standard, a choice must be made between setting an *absolute* standard of performance or adopting a *relative* standard. An absolute standard is one which requires that examinees answer some predetermined number or percentage of questions correctly to pass the examination. A relative standard, on the other hand, is one in which the pass/fail level is determined by selecting a point on the distribution curve of some group of examinees who have taken the test.

Absolute standards for certification of physicians have great appeal on emotional grounds. One would like to believe that there is some absolutely minimal amount of knowledge, depth of understanding and degree of skill which every physician must have achieved before he is permitted to practice medicine, even in the confines of a teaching hospital under the close supervision of resident and attending staff. But how much knowledge is enough? To what degree must he understand? Exactly how skillful must he be?

Efforts have been made to set absolute standards for achievement tests in medicine. In grading essay examinations, for example, the examiner frequently has some idea regarding the minimum amount of information that must be supplied by the examinee in order to "pass" an individual question or the examination as a whole.

A method for attempting to set an absolute standard for an objective test, proposed by Nedelsky[11] in 1954, has been used by some medical schools and at least one specialty board.[12] In this procedure a "minimum passing level" (MPL) is determined for each individual test item, these MPLs are summed for all items, and the resulting overall MPL is adjusted by an arbitrarily chosen constant to arrive at the standard for passing the examination. To arrive at an MPL for each item, the examiner must first define a minimally acceptable student and then decide which of the answers to each test question would be recognized as wrong by minimally acceptable students but not by unacceptable students. This procedure appears to be similar to asking the examiner to predict the difficulty level of each individual test question, for a subsample of the examinee group, without benefit of previous performance statistics for the questions. Moreover, if the resulting standards are to be fair to all examinees, examiners must be consistent from subject to subject and from year to year in deciding upon MPLs. Otherwise, standards may fluctuate in an unpredictable fashion and examinees who fail may well have a legitimate complaint about the capriciousness of the certification system.

While the MPL is emotionally appealing, one must question whether examiners can make such predictions with a high degree of reliability and validity, and whether the resulting standards can have the stability required for an instrument that is to be used for purposes of certification.

Attempting to set an absolute standard for examination performance is an extremely difficult task, even when the test is limited to a particular course in a particular medical school taught by the same individual who creates the examination. Therefore, it is not surprising that the medical educators who construct National Board examinations find it impossible to set absolute standards for these tests, which cover fairly broad areas of medical knowledge and will be taken by students with a wide variety of educational experiences.

Relative standards achieve stability of failure rates from subject to subject and from year to year if these standards are based upon the performance of fairly large reference groups the "quality" of which is stable over time. For National Board examinations, reference groups are defined as all students at a specified level of training (second year for Part I, fourth year for Part II) who are taking the examination for the first time and who are taking it as candidates for National Board certification. These reference groups now number several thousand students annually for each Part of the examination.

The minimum passing score for Part I is set at 1.2 standard deviation units below the mean of this reference group. This minimum passing level corresponds to a standard score of 380 and yields a failure rate of approximately 10 per cent for the Part I reference group. The minimum passing score for Part II and Part III is set at 2.1 standard deviation units below the mean of the Part II and Part III reference groups respectively. On the standard score scale, this minimum passing score is a score of 290, yielding a failure rate of approximately 2 per cent for each of these reference groups.

Each of the three Parts of the National Board examinations is now administered twice a year. Because the Board uses a relative approach to standard setting, it is important to establish a mechanism whereby the same standard is set for each of these two test administrations even if the groups of examinees who are tested are not comparable. The examinee groups taking Part I in September, in contrast to those taking Part I in June, generally are not representative of all medical students at that level of education and score somewhat less well than the June examinees. However, scores on the September test must be comparable to those reported for the June administration if the same minimum passing score is to be used for both tests.

The procedure used for equating June and September scores is to compare the performance of previous June and current September examinees on questions from previous June examinations which are embedded in the current September test. With this comparison in hand, the September scores may be equated with those expected of June examinees on that particular September test.

Recent experience with the April and September administrations of the Part II examination has indicated that the two examinee groups are comparable. Therefore, a separate reference group has been identified for each administration of Part II and no formal equating of scores is necessary.

For Part III, candidates who take the test in May generally perform less well than those who are tested in March. Therefore, as with Part I, scores from the May administration of Part II are equated with those from the March administration in order to achieve a common standard for the two tests.

The major argument advanced by critics of relative standards is that the population of examinees upon which the standards are based may change—either suddenly as a result of new and different kinds of individuals introduced into the system, or gradually as a result of evolutionary processes within the system. Therefore, the argument continues, if an examination system imposes a fixed failure rate, individuals who would have failed in the past may now pass the test or vice versa, depending upon the direction in which the examinee population has shifted.

This argument fails to consider a number of important factors that can alter this apparently inevitable conclusion. First, it is unlikely that the competence of the large mass of medical students will show any drastic change, either upward or downward, in a relatively short period of time. Thus, in the short run, when a large percentage of the student population is included in the reference group a relative standard should be at least as stable as an absolute standard.

Second, it appears that in the long run the performance expected of the student is related to the quality of students electing medicine as a career and to the quality of the medical education they receive. Many educators believe that the student of today is better prepared, more highly motivated and more able intellectually than the student of 20 years ago, and that the medical educational system of today is substantially better than it was in the past. However, the level of expectation, in an absolute sense, also appears to be greater than it was in the past. Many would not now be satisfied with a performance considered minimally acceptable 20 years ago.

In addition, it is necessary to consider the effect of an absolute standard upon the educational system itself. If an absolute standard were established, the educational system would undoubtedly attempt to gear its selection mechanisms and teaching programs to meet this standard. In time, and at some cost, any reasonable standard probably would be surpassed by all but a very few individuals, and the failure rate for the certification process would approach zero. As this would occur, the motivational value of certification would diminish.

In spite of these counterarguments, major changes in the performance of a reference group, if they occurred and were not detected, would pose a serious problem for a system which uses a relative standard. Therefore, in recent years the National Board has developed a technique for monitoring the stability of its reference groups from year to year. We have called this technique the "test-within-a-test" since its essential feature is the inclusion of a set of test items which have appeared in recent previous National Board examinations into each new examination, balancing the content of these used questions according to the same content outline used for the whole examination. This test-within-a-test is then used to monitor reference-group performance. Each year the performance of previous reference groups on these questions is estimated from item statistics and compared with the performance of the current reference group. Since the questions are the same, any significant difference in performance may be attributed to a difference between the current and previous reference groups.

The results for the June 1972 through 1976 Part I examinations indicate that current reference groups are scoring slightly higher than previous groups on the same questions. The difference in mean scores on the total examination is from one to two percentage points. There is no indication of a trend toward lower performance in any of the subjects. These data, therefore, indicate that the standard for passing Part I is not eroding. If any change is occurring, the Part I standard appears to be increasing slightly with time. Analyses reviewed to date based on similar procedures for the Part II examination suggest a similar conclusion for that examination.

To the time of this writing, the National Board has decided not to change its standards on the basis of this information since the shift in reference-group performance has been very slight and has been in the direction of maintaining a high standard for National Board certification. The process (or an improved version of it) will continue to be used to monitor reference-group performance in future examinations, and the results of these analyses, together with other relevant information, will be reviewed regularly by the Board in judging the appropriateness of its standards and in deciding whether or not changes in those standards should be made. In the end, any standard-setting procedure must inevitably rely on human judgment. It is essential, however, that such judgment be based upon as much relevant information (both statistical and nonstatistical) as can be obtained. Over the years, the National Board has been keenly aware of its responsibility for setting standards that are realistic in terms of the high quality of medical education offered in the United States, but it is also aware of the fact that some students (hopefully very few) are not ready for certification at the time they take these examinations. In addition, the Board is mindful of the fact that standards should not be "set in concrete," but that change must be made deliberately rather than allowed to occur in a capricious manner. As stated by Dr. Robert Ebel[13] ". . . a variety of approaches can be used to solve the problem of defining the passing score. Unfortunately, different approaches are likely to give different results. Anyone who expects to discover the 'real' passing score by any of these approaches, or any other approach, is doomed to disappointment, for a 'real' passing score does not exist to be discovered. All any examining authority that must set passing scores can hope for, and all any of their examinees can ask, is that the basis for defining the passing scored be defined clearly, and that the definition be as rational as possible."

References

1. Spearman, C.: Coefficient of correlation calculated from faulty data. Br. J. Psychol., 3:271, 1910.
2. Hoyt, C.: Test reliability estimated by analysis of variance. Psychometrica, 6:153, 1941.
3. Jackson, R. W. B.: Reliability of mental tests. Br. J. Psychol., 29:267, 1939.
4. Richardson, M. W., and Kuder, F.: The calculation of test-reliability coefficients based upon the method of rational equivalence. J. Educ. Psychol., 30:681, 1939.
5. Kuder, G. R. and Richardson, M. W.: The theory of estimation of test reliability. Psychometrica, 2:151, 1937.
6. Swineford, F.: Some relations between test scores and item statistics. J. Educ. Psychol., 50:26, 1959.
7. Levit, E. J. (Ed.): Report of the Policy Advisory Committee of the National Board of Medical Examiners (Holden, W. D., Chairman). National Board of Medical Examiners, Philadelphia, 1976.
8. Cowles, J. T. and Hubbard, J. P.: A comparative study of essay and objective examinations for medical students. J. Med. Educ., 27(Part 2):14, 1952.
9. Cowles, J. T. and Hubbard, J. P.: Validity and reliability of the new objective tests. J. Med. Educ., 29(6):30, 1954.
10. Hubbard, J. P. and Cowles, J. T.: A comparative study of student performance in medical schools using National Board examinations. J. Med. Educ., 29(7):27, 1954.
11. Nedelsky, L.: Absolute grading standards for objective tests. Educ. Psychol. Meas., 14:3, 1954.
12. Levine, H. G. and McGuire, C.: Use of profile system for scoring and reporting certifying examinations in orthopedic surgery. J. Med. Educ., 46:78, 1971.
13. Ebel, R. L.: Essentials of Educational Measurement. Prentice-Hall, Englewood Cliffs, 1972.

CHAPTER 7

■

Results of Examinations Reported to Medical Schools

Each year the deans of medical schools receive confidential memoranda reporting the performance of their student classes on National Board examinations. Quite obviously these reports apply only to schools in which an appreciable number of students take the examinations. Where a relatively small proportion of a class is included in the examinations, average scores have little value for judging the performance of the class in one major subject in comparison with its performance in other subjects, or for comparing mean scores of the class with mean scores of the national population of National Board candidates.

A report of the results of the Part I examination for 1976 is included here as an example of the amount and type of information routinely made available to medical school faculties; a similar report is distributed annually for the Part II examination. Another report is prepared for the Part III examination so that medical schools may see how their graduates performed at a clinical level one year after graduation. For all schools receiving these reports, detailed information is made available to indicate how one student class compared with the national averages. Thus, medical school faculties may judge, on the basis of precise, objective examinations, how well or how poorly their students handled the comprehensive examinations and the several categories for which subscores are reported.

Candidates and Noncandidates

There is a considerable and consistent difference between the performances of candidates (those who elect to register as candidates for ultimate National Board certification, irrespective of whether the examination is a requirement of their medical schools) and noncandidates (students who take the examination only as a requirement of their medical schools). The candidates invariably have mean scores higher than those of the noncandidates. Among the factors that may lie behind this difference are the attitudes toward the examinations of both students and faculty. If students are required to take National Board examinations without much forewarning, and are assured that the results will in no way affect their school grades or their standings in their classes, they may have little motivation to do well. Knowing that they may derive no personal benefit from them, they may have casual or even antagonistic attitudes toward the examinations. Under these circumstances the results cannot be compared fairly with those in which students are trying to do their best. The results are meaningless and may even be misleading.

In addition to motivational factors, it is likely that some of the difference between candidates and noncandidates is due to a self-selection process. Because the decision to take examinations for National Board credit is largely in the hands of the individual student (even though a school may require him to take the tests), it is reasonable to assume that those students confident of passing are more likely to take the tests for credit than are those less sure of their ability to do well. The less confident students may be tempted to take their chances with state board examinations at a later date. In some schools where Part I or Part II grades count heavily in determining final class grades (i.e., where students are highly motivated), significant differences in test performance still occur between the candidate and noncandidate groups. In this situation it appears that self-selection in the candidate group, rather than motivational factors, explains the difference in performance.

Too Much Reliance on National Boards

Prior to the introduction of multiple-choice techniques in the examinations of the National Board, faculties of medical schools had to rely upon their own assessments of their students' acquisition of medical knowledge. When the results of reliable extramural examinations became available, a new instrument for educational measurement was accessible to the medical faculties. Those who were members of National Board test committees brought to their faculty colleagues an awareness of the objectivity, validity and reliability of these examinations. Extramural measurements were introduced as comprehensive evaluations of students at periodic points along the four-year course (Part I usually at the end of the second year and Part II near the end of the fourth year). An increasing number of department chairmen elected to substitute National Board examinations for in-course tests and also for final departmental examinations. The instrument intended to be a useful aid to faculties in judging their students had, in some instances, become the sole determinant of student advancement and even graduation.

The National Board has frequently expressed its disapproval of such use—or misuse—of the results of its examinations but has not considered it appropriate to become involved in the intramural policies of any medical school. Test scores derived from extramural examinations may be useful in appraising student performance, but were never intended to relieve faculty of its own responsibility in making periodic or final judgments about its students.

Report of a Part I Examination

Following is an example of a report of the Part I examination combining the two administrations in June and September of 1976. As shown in Table 1, this examination was taken by a total of 9,683 examinees with 8,647 having signed up as candidates and 1,036 as noncandidates taking the examination only as a requirement of their medical schools.

Great emphasis is placed upon maintaining the confidential nature of the information contained in these annual reports. The performance of the students of each school is made available only to that school and is not released to any other school or agency. With this information in hand, the school may, if it wishes, compare the performance of its students with that of the total population of students taking this examination. In the tables the designation "your school" refers to the school that receives the report pertaining to its own students.

Table 1 shows the performance of all second-year examinees (candidates and noncandidates separately) on each Part I subject and the total test. The data included are mean scores, standard deviations, pass rates for the total population and pass rates for the students of that school ("your school"). The minimum standard score required to pass Part I in 1976 was a score of 380 on the total test. Minimum passing scores for individual subjects are not established by the National Board.

Table 2 shows graphically how "your students" performed in relation to the National Board candidate group in one of the subtests of Part I (biochemistry) and on the total test. Similar data are reported for each of the seven subjects that constitute the total Part I examination. This table, in addition to the bar graphs, contains the following statistical information for the candidate group and for "your students" for the designated subtests:

1. Number of examinees
2. Average scores for the group
3. Range within which the average score for the group would be expected to fall by chance alone with odds of 2 to 1 ($\pm$ 1 standard error of the mean)
4. Per cent of the group falling below the candidate group average
5. Standard deviation for the group

The graphic display on this table consists of two computer-generated bar charts superimposed on the same axes. The chart drawn by using the letter X shows the performance of the total candidate group, while the chart drawn with the letter O shows the performance of "your students."

In these displays, the abscissa (horizontal axis) is a standard score scale shown in 25-point intervals, while the ordinate (vertical axis) is the percentage of an examinee group. Each individual X or O represents 0.5 per cent of its corresponding group. Thus, each X bar and O bar shows the percentage of the candidate group and the percentage of "your students," respectively, that fell into each 25-point score interval on a given Part I subject or on the total test. The highest percentage listed on the ordinate is 20 per cent. If a school should have more than 20 per cent of its students in a particular score interval, the topmost O is replaced by a number giving the actual per cent.

The standard score scale (horizontal axis) of the charts shows the lowest and highest scores obtained by any examinee in the National Board candidate group. The first bars show the percentage of the candidate group and the percentage of "your students" who scored between the lowest score and a score

Table 1.   Performance of Second-year Candidates, Noncandidates and Your Students on the June and September 1976 Part I Examination

	School		School Code	
	Candidates (Number = 8647)		Noncandidates (Number = 1036)	
Subject	Mean	S.D.	Mean	S.D.
Anatomy	500	100	484	107
Physiology	501	99	482	104
Biochemistry	500	99	477	105
Pathology	500	99	466	112
Microbiology	500	99	465	106
Pharmacology	500	100	472	116
Behavioral Science	500	100	483	103
Total Test	500	99	470	111

Per cent passing (total test score = 380 or above)

	Candidates		Noncandidates		Total	
	N	Per cent pass	N	Per cent pass	N	Per cent pass
All examinees	8,647	89.1	1,036	80.6	9,683	88.2
Your school	130	85.4	0	.0	130	85.4

Table 2. Performance of Second-year NBME Candidates and Your Students Part I Examinations (June and September 1976)

Biochemistry

School		School code
Candidate group = X		Your students = O
Number = 8647		Number = 130
Average score = 500		Average score = 455
Chance range of average score = 499–501		Chance range of average score = 448–462
Per cent below average score = 49%		Per cent below candidate group average = 67%
Standard deviation = 99		Standard deviation = 83

```
Per Cent of Examinees

20 ───────────────────────────────────────────────────────

19

18 ───────────────────────────────────────────────────────

17

16 ───────────────────────────────────────────────────────

15

14 ───────────────────────────────────────────────────────

13

12 ───────────────────────────────────────────────────────
                    O   O
11                  O   O  X            X
                    O   O  X            X
10              O   O   O  XO       O  XO
                    O   O   O  XO       O  XO
 9                  O   O   O  XO   O   O  XO
                    O   O   O  XO  XO  XO  XO
 8                  O   O   O  XO  XO  XO  XO
                    O   O   O  XO  XO  XO  XO  X
 7                  O   O  XO  XO  XO  XO  XO  XO      X
                    O   O  XO  XO  XO  XO  XO  XO  X   X
 6                  O  XO  XO  XO  XO  XO  XO  XO  X   X
               XO  XO  XO  XO  XO  XO  XO  XO  X   X
 5             XO  XO  XO  XO  XO  XO  XO  XO  X   X
          O    XO  XO  XO  XO  XO  XO  XO  XO  X   X
 4        O   O   O  XO  XO  XO  XO  XO  XO  XO  X   X   X
          O   O  XO  XO  XO  XO  XO  XO  XO  XO  X   X   X
 3        O   O  XO  XO  XO  XO  XO  XO  XO  XO  XO X   X   X
          O  XO  XO  XO  XO  XO  XO  XO  XO  XO  XO X   X   X
 2       XO  XO  XO  XO  XO  XO  XO  XO  XO  XO  XO XO X   X   X   X
     O       XO  XO  XO  XO  XO  XO  XO  XO  XO  XO XO X  XO X   X
 1   O  XO  XO  XO  XO  XO  XO  XO  XO  XO  XO  XO  XO XO XO XO X   X
   X  XO  XO  XO  XO  XO  XO  XO  XO  XO  XO  XO  XO XO XO XO XO X  X   X
```

| 135 | 250 | 275 | 300 | 325 | 350 | 375 | 400 | 425 | 450 | 475 | 500 | 525 | 550 | 575 | 600 | 625 | 650 | 675 | 700 | 725 | 750 |
| 245 | 270 | 295 | 320 | 345 | 370 | 395 | 420 | 445 | 470 | 495 | 520 | 545 | 570 | 595 | 620 | 645 | 670 | 695 | 720 | 745 | 825 |

Standard score

Per cent below											
candidate group	1	2	7	16	29	49	68	82	93	98	100
Your school	0	2	11	25	48	67	87	97	99	100	100

of 245. Similarly, the last bars show the percentage of these groups that scored between 750 and the highest score obtained.

The two rows of numbers at the bottom of the chart show the percentage of the candidate group and the percentage of "your students" that fell below each 50-point interval on the standard score scale (i.e., below 250, 300, 350, etc.). These two percentages (which are actually percentile standings) provide another means for comparing "your students" with the candidate group.

CHAPTER 8

■

Qualifying Examinations Derived from Standardized Test Material

The National Board's collection of test questions, used and calibrated against standards of medical education throughout the United States, provides a resource that is drawn upon as a basis for setting standards for an increasing number of examination programs. Since precise information is available to identify the difficulty of each question and its ability to discriminate between the more competent and the less competent examinees, an examination made up of such questions can be related to standards that are current and sensitive to the dynamic nature of medical education throughout the United States.

Among those drawing upon this resource are the Federation of State Medical Boards, the Educational Commission for Foreign Medical Graduates and the Medical Council of Canada. Most recently the National Board has responded to the federal government to provide an examination to meet certain requirements placed upon immigrating alien physicians.

Federation Licensing Examination (FLEX)

The Background for FLEX

Despite early apprehension about the institution of a "national" qualifying examination and its relationship to the legally constituted licensing authorities of the states,[1,2] the state boards themselves came to recognize the advantages and superior quality of the National Board's multiple-choice examinations. In 1953, soon after the Board's change-over from essay examinations, Connecticut was the first state to request the National Board to provide examinations to be administered under state law in place of essay examinations prepared and graded by its own board of examiners. The move was well received. The state board had an external criterion, i.e., the performance of medical students and graduates throughout the United States, against which to judge the performance of its own candidates, many of whom were graduates of foreign medical schools. The idea spread to other states, especially those with large numbers of candidates; New York, Massachusetts, Virginia and Illinois soon followed Connecticut's lead.

Over the course of several years, an increasing number of states elected to take this route to a higher quality of licensing examination. Concurrently the Federation of State Medical Boards sought, through a series of examination institutes, to achieve greater uniformity of standards for medical licensure while, at the same time, preserving the constitutional right of each state to regulate and control the practice of medicine within its borders. In 1967, the Federation's Examination Institute Committee, expressing an earnest desire to move constructively toward its declared objective of uniform standards for determining qualification for a medical license, sought the assistance of the National Board. By this time the Board was providing approximately 25,000 tests annually for 16 state boards for the examination of about 3,000 physicians. The trend was well established.

These two developments—the increasing use of test questions derived from the National Board's standardized pool of material and the determination of the Federation's Examination Institute Committee to achieve a higher quality of state-board examinations—led to an agreement between the National Board and the Federation for the development of a Federation Licensing Examination (FLEX), the objective of which was to place state medical licensing examinations and procedures in definite relationship to modern medical education with special emphasis upon the clinical competence of candidates for a state license. The acceptance of the FLEX examination by the individual state boards grew more rapidly than even its most optimistic proponents anticipated. Within a period of about ten years this examination had been generally accepted by state boards in their requirements for a medical license.

The Examination

A test committee of members of state boards meets regularly with the staff of the National Board to design and construct the examination. The members of this committee are responsible for selecting the questions according to their collective judgment as to the appropriateness of each item for candidates for a state license. As the committee members know from experience in their own states, many of these candidates have graduated from medical school many years earlier, many of them will have had backgrounds with widely differing standards and curricula and many may be unfamiliar with much that is to be found in the current pool of National Board test material, especially in the basic medical sciences. The committee, therefore, gives careful attention to the relevance of each question for the current practice of medicine.

The examination extends over three days. The first day includes seven basic medical science areas, providing 80 test items in each subject. The basic-science subjects are: anatomy, behavioral sciences, biochemistry, microbiology, pathology, pharmacology and physiology. The items are arranged in multidisciplinary form so that the subject-matter origin of an individual item is not identified. The second day includes six clinical-science areas, with 90 test items in each subject. The clinical-science subjects are: internal medicine, obstetrics and gynecology, pediatrics, preventive medicine and public health, psychiatry and surgery, including items in medical jurisprudence. These items, too, are presented in multidisciplinary form.

The third day of the test contains test material drawn from the National Board's Part III examination. It includes clinical material presented in the form of pictures of patients, gross and microscopic specimens, roentgenograms, electrocardiograms, charts and tables, about which searching questions are asked. A distinctive feature of the third day is the programmed testing based upon patient management problems, to assess the candidate's judgment in the sequential management of clinical problems similar to those encountered in day-to-day practice (see Chapter 4).

The scoring of the FLEX examination is done by the National Board and is related directly to the performance of National Board candidates as determined by the item analysis of the test questions. Since the difficulty of each item (the P value) and the index of discrimination (r_{bis}) are known for each item, an accurate estimate may be made of the scores that would be expected for National Board candidates if they were to take the FLEX examination.

Although each of the three sections of the examination is set up and presented to the candidates in multidisciplinary form, without identification of its component subjects (i.e., as a scrambled examination), a score is derived for each major subject in order to satisfy state laws and regulations. Many states require numeric scores in specified subjects, most often in terms of 75 per cent for a minimum passing level. (One wonders about the origin of the 75 per cent level, and even more about the meaning of 75 per cent of the knowledge of a subject such as internal medicine. The only possible explanation is that this minimal level is traditional. At any rate, the tradition persists to the extent that the FLEX examination scores are reported so that a scale score of 75 can be accepted by state boards as a legally authorized minimum passing level.)

The first step in scoring FLEX is to obtain scores for each of the subjects of the basic medical science section (Day 1), each of the clinical subjects (Day 2) and the clinical competence section (Day 3). The subject scores for Day 1 are then averaged to give a comprehensive score for the basic medical sciences. Similarly, the subject scores for the second day are averaged to provide a comprehensive score for the clinical sciences. A weighted average is then determined so as to give major emphasis to clinical competence. The scoring formula gives the basic-science section (the first day) a weight of one, the clinical-science section (the second day) a weight of two and the test of clinical competence (the third day) a weight of three. This weighted average is reported to the Federation together with the scores on individual subjects and average scores for the basic medical sciences, the clinical subjects and clinical competence. The Federation in turn transmits these scores to the individual states. Although each state has the right to interpret the scores in accordance with its own laws and regulations, the FLEX weighted average has become the final determinant of passing or failing irrespective of the scores on individual subjects and independent also of the one-day averages for basic sciences, clinical subjects or clinical competence. Thus the scoring method adopted by the FLEX Committee acknowledges the responsibility of state licensing boards in determining the qualification of physicians who have graduated from medical school, who have had supervised responsibility for the care of patients in a hospital as interns or residents and who may have had additional years of clinical experience before registering for the FLEX examination.

FLEX and the National Board Examinations: A Dual System

Now that the FLEX program has become established and its examination accepted by all state licensing boards, a dual examination system has evolved in the United States. Almost all students in American medical schools choose to take Parts I and II of the National Board examinations as they progress through their formal medical school years, finishing with Part III during or after the first year in hospital residency. A diminishing few students opt to wait and take the three-day FLEX examination during or after the first year of graduate training, although realizing that by so doing they may encounter an embarrassing delay in licensure in the event of failure. The FLEX examinations (19,975 in 1977) are, therefore, taken predominantly by graduates of foreign medical schools who are not eligible for admission to the National Board examinations.

This dual system is a point that continues to need clarification. The examiners of the National Board (the members of its several test committees) are charged with the responsibility of formulating examinations to test the knowledge of students as they are learning medicine in medical school today. This objective is different from that of evaluating competence to practice medicine for individuals who may be some years removed from their formal courses in areas such as biochemistry or anatomy. Since the objectives are different, the examinations should be different—each aimed at its own clearly defined target.

Thus, an entirely logical dual system has developed: the National Board examinations focused upon the student of today who is the physician of tomorrow, and the FLEX examination to assess the knowledge and more especially the clinical competence of the physician of today who was the student of earlier years.

Examinations for the Medical Council of Canada

Closely related to the use of the National Board's collection of examination material for FLEX and licensure in the United States has been for several years a similar use of this collection of pretested standardized questions for the Medical Council of Canada and official licensure in Canada. Here again a multidisciplinary committee appointed by the Council has been meeting annually with the medical and psychometric staff of the National Board to formulate an examination according to specifications drawn up by the Council and in keeping with medical education in Canada. These examinations, containing multiple-choice questions in clinical areas and patient management problems, are very similar to the National Board's Part II and Part III examinations. An additional feature of the program is a translation into French for this bilingual nation.

After some ten years of close cooperation between the Medical Council of Canada and the National Board of Medical Examiners in the formulation of the qualifying examinations accepted by all Canadian provinces, the Canadian Council, not unreasonably, came to the conclusion that it should gradually effect a well-considered phasing out of reliance upon the National Board of Medical Examiners and assume full responsibility for its own examinations itself.

The ECFMG Examination

Another testing program depending upon the National Board's pool of standardized, pretested multiple-choice questions is that of the Educational Commission for Foreign Medical Graduates (ECFMG). This program was initiated in 1958 for the primary purpose of determining, on an individual basis, whether a graduate of a medical school outside of the United States or Canada could be considered sufficiently well qualified to serve as intern or resident in an American hospital, to assume supervised responsibility for the care and well-being of patients and to profit from an opportunity for graduate medical education in the United States. Before this time, the American Medical Association with the cooperation of the Association of American Medical Colleges had published a list of foreign schools, the graduates of which could be considered on an equal basis with graduates of medical schools in the United States. It soon became apparent, however, that the point of real concern was not so much the caliber of the school from which the individual had been graduated as the caliber of the individual himself.

Accordingly, agreement was reached to establish a testing procedure to permit direct comparison between the medical knowledge of any graduate of any recognized medical school in the world* and that of graduates of medical schools in the United States and Canada. To achieve this objective, the ECFMG turned to the National Board and its large collection of questions, for each of which the level of difficulty and index of discrimination are known from previous testing of American students. By careful selection of questions and appropriate scoring procedures, examinations are prepared so that the scores for those taking the ECFMG examination are derived from the scores that would have been received by a National Board examinee.

Although the passing score for the ECFMG examination is again the traditional 75, it must not be assumed that passing the ECFMG examination is equivalent to passing National Board examinations. To achieve certification by the National Board, a candidate must successfully complete a total of five days of examination. The ECFMG examination is completed in one day and, on this one day, six and one-half hours are allowed for the number of questions that would have been allowed four and one-half hours on National Boards. Questions previously used in National Board examinations are carefully selected with emphasis on those elements of medical knowledge generally applicable on a worldwide basis. As noted above, the initial purpose of the ECFMG examination was to serve as a test of qualification for appointment as intern or resident in an American hospital, working under supervision. Certification by the National Board, on the other hand, is regarded as qualification for licensure for the independent practice of medicine.

The ECFMG examinations are all in the English language; it would be impossible to translate them into the many languages of the examinees. Furthermore, the basic purpose of the examination is to determine an individual's qualification for an appointment in an American hospital where he communicates with American physicians and American patients in English.

---

* "A recognized medical school" was defined as any medical school listed in the Directory of Medical Schools published by the World Health Organization (Geneva, 1963).

Consequently, a test of the physician's comprehension of the English language is included among the requirements for certification by the ECFMG.*

Through the mechanisms detailed above, the United States thus opened the doorway to graduates of foreign medical schools for graduate education as interns or residents in American hospitals. The intent of the program was to provide an experience in graduate medical education extending over two or three years, after which these individuals would return to their homelands having benefited from this opportunity. Had the program developed according to this worthy intent, it might well have been viewed as a significant contribution of American medicine to nations where the need was great.

Things did not, however, work out as had been anticipated. The doorway, having been opened, attracted a rapidly increasing stream of physicians of varying competence and quality. In 1965 the doorway was opened further by an amendment to the Immigration and Nationality Act whereby physicians were given preference for immigration visas whether or not they had been certified by the ECFMG.

As shown in Table 2, Chapter 1, the number of ECFMG examinations administered annually between the years 1960 to 1976 leveled off at about 30,000 in over 150 designated foreign centers at home and around the world. Within this total number, there were many taking the examination repetitively after initial failures; the failures on the examination usually averaged 40 to 50 per cent of the number at any single administration. Of those who passed and came to the United States, an uncounted number were to be found taking part in hospital and community services with or without appropriate supervision. In 1976, a total of 29,495 ECFMG examinations was administered, predominantly to foreign medical graduates, and of this number 43 per cent failed. During this year (1976), 35 per cent of a total of 16,859 newly licensed physicians entering practice in the United States were graduates of foreign medical schools.

The failure rate of foreign physicians on the licensing examination for independent practice administered by the states (FLEX) has also remained high. Little has been known about the role in medical care of those who failed the FLEX examination and thereby did not obtain licenses.[3]

The Visa Qualifying Examination (VQE)

Out of this background, the federal government stepped into the situation and called for more stringent screening procedures *before* an alien medical graduate could obtain a visa to enter the United States. The Health Professions Educational Assistance Act of 1976 required the passing of Parts I and II of the National Board examinations or "an equivalent examination as determined by the Secretary of Health, Education, and Welfare." Since it was the long-standing policy of the National Board that alien graduates of foreign medical schools are not eligible for its Part I and Part II examinations, agreement was reached to take the alternative course offered by the new legislation to provide "an equivalent examination." The ECFMG examination, even if altered, having

---

* An informational booklet is published by the Educational Commission for Foreign Medical Graduates, 3624 Market Street, Philadelphia, Pennsylvania 19104, USA.

been considered unacceptable for this purpose by the government, the National Board decided that, in the public interest, it should generate a special examination which for the purposes of the law could be considered equivalent to Part I and Part II of the National Board examinations. This examination became known as the Visa Qualifying Examination (VQE).

The VQE was constructed as a two-day examination composed of items from regular National Board examinations. Although it is only half as long as the standard Part I and Part II, the content of each of its categories is strictly comparable to that of the corresponding category of the regular examinations. It is made up of 900 to 1,000 questions in multiple-choice form and is given only in the English language. About half of the questions are drawn in equal numbers from the basic-science disciplines of anatomy, behavioral sciences, biochemistry, microbiology, pathology, pharmacology and physiology and the remaining half of the questions are drawn equally from the clinical sciences of internal medicine, obstetrics and gynecology, pediatrics, preventive medicine and public health, psychiatry and surgery.

Scoring is standardized directly on the performance of the identical questions in the National Board examinations taken by American medical students. The basic-science and the clinical-science sections must each be passed as separate sections under scoring standards identical to those applying to the National Board's Parts I and II. Because of the abbreviated length of the examination, no subscores for individual subjects are derived and the examinee's achievement is recorded as pass or fail on each section of the examination.

Public Law 94-484 also requires that alien physicians applying for visas must be proficient in the English language. Consequently, the National Board is requiring that this proficiency be demonstrated prior to taking the VQE. Therefore, to be eligible for the VQE, the candidate must meet English requirements specified by the ECFMG within two years prior to taking the VQE. The only other prerequisite is satisfactory evidence of graduation from a medical school listed by the World Health Organization.

While offering the VQE to comply with the requirements of Public Law 94-484, the National Board nevertheless has been concerned about certain aspects of its application. The examination must attempt an assessment of the educational content of four years of the medical curriculum in a single two-day period because of the specification that applicants must be graduates of a medical school. This specification precludes the customary opportunity given American students to take the basic-science portion separately and well before graduation. The VQE is a rigorous examination, the content of which may not be as attuned to native curricula as it is to the American curricula. In the introduction of the examination, the National Board anticipated a high failure rate; this anticipation was fulfilled by the fact that the failure rate on the first examination administered in September 1977 was 75 per cent.

References

1. Derbyshire, R. C.: *Medical Licensure and Discipline in the United States.* The Johns Hopkins Press, Baltimore, 1969.
2. Shryock, R. H.: *Medical Licensing in America, 1650—1965.* The Johns Hopkins Press, Baltimore, 1967.
3. *Physician Distribution and Licensure in the U.S., 1975.* American Medical Association, Chicago, 1976.

CHAPTER 9

■

Evaluation as a Guide to Learning in Graduate and Continuing Education*

During medical school a student undergoes a variety of objective and subjective judgments made by the faculty as well as episodic examination procedures designed to determine his qualification for a course grade, for promotion to the next class or for graduation and an M.D. degree. These may be faculty-made examinations or the extramural examinations of the National Board. At the graduate level the physician must take and pass examinations of the specialty board in his chosen field if he wishes to be certified as a specialist. All of these examinations have one feature in common: that of determining individual competence or qualification at a specific point in preparation for a career in medicine. This common feature identifies examinations as qualifying examinations, measuring the product of the educational system.

Examinations also serve as guides to learning during the course of the learning process, and therefore become part of the learning process. Careful analysis of examination results provides specific information to the educator relative to teaching, and to the educatee relative to learning.

Evaluation of Learning at the Graduate Level

Whereas evaluation of learning has been well established during the formal years of undergraduate medical education, similar ongoing evaluation at the graduate level has more recently gained attention and increasing application. To be sure, the program director and others on the staff of a teaching hospital can and do evaluate the competence and skill of the resident in the day-to-day exchange in the clinic, at the bedside and in the conference room. Because of its nature, however, graduate education as conducted in a clinical setting poses certain limitations with respect to evaluation of learning.

Learning at the graduate level is characteristically independent. As the resident assumes increasing responsibility for patient care and also for his own

---

* *Graduate* as used in this text refers to internship and residency; *continuing medical education* refers to the continuing lifelong career of the physician.

continuing education, the program director has less and less opportunity to observe and to evaluate the progress and learning that may or may not have taken place.

Also, since in most residency programs the resident rotates through related disciplines, the program director cannot always assess the effectiveness of these experiences. He must sometimes depend upon the judgment of those outside the specialty for evaluation of trainee learning.

As a result of these educational variables, all of which limit the evaluation process, basic deficiencies in the learning of the individual trainee may go undetected during the training period.

Following residency training, one or more years of practice experience may be required before a physician is eligible for certification by a specialty board. Such practice experience is relatively unstructured and, therefore, allows for wide variations in the type and quality of learning that may take place. Many years may elapse between the time a physician embarks upon his graduate training and the "moment of truth" when he is confronted by the examination of his specialty board. This examination, intended primarily as a qualifying examination, can come too late in his career to provide a useful learning experience.

One of the most disturbing aspects of the training and certifying procedure in graduate medical education has been the high failure rates sometimes encountered for those who have completed approved training programs extending over five to seven years and have met all the requirements for the examination.

Since all candidates have been trained in approved programs, have been considered qualified by their respective program directors and have met all eligibility requirements, these high failure rates are indeed difficult to understand. It would, of course, be naive to assume that all approved programs are of comparable quality, or that all individuals entering these training programs are of comparable caliber. Even in the face of these variations in quality, however, why are so many individuals so poorly prepared by the time they reach the certifying examination? What factors account for these failure rates? Is the certifying examination itself at fault? Is the quantity or the quality of graduate training deficient? Do program directors accept and approve trainees who are inadequate in caliber or poorly suited to the specialty concerned?

In-training Examination for Residents as a Guide to Learning

Seriously concerned about the high percentage of presumably carefully selected and well-trained candidates who failed to pass its qualifying examination after seven or more years of training, the American Board of Neurological Surgery undertook to study its educational programs and qualifying examination.[1-6] In 1962, the Board appointed a commission under the auspices of the American Association of Neurological Surgeons (the Harvey Cushing Society) to study the problem.[2] The objective was to develop a program to improve the quality and effectiveness of residency training in neurosurgery as well as the preparation of individual candidates for certification, and hence to increase the competence of all those entering the specialty.

Various measures were considered. The possibility of giving an aptitude test at the end of the year of internship, before accepting a trainee for specialty training, seemed unrealistic and of questionable value. The possibility of encouraging each program director to conduct an examination of his own every year or two during the training period was considered to have merit, but variable and impractical to implement.

The possibility of conducting a uniform examination during the period of formal training seemed to be theoretically most desirable and likely to provide useful information about both the caliber of the trainee and the quality of the training program. More specifically, the introduction of an in-training examination could, it was hoped, identify areas of weakness in the knowledge of the trainee or deficiencies in the training program itself, so that trainees and their program directors could then endeavor to correct these weaknesses during the course of the training period.

The commission and the officers of the Board of Neurological Surgery met with the staff of the National Board. Many aspects of the plan were discussed, the objectives of the program were reviewed and an outline of an examination was drawn up to meet the stated objectives. A multiple-choice examination was developed to measure knowledge and comprehension of those areas of neurosurgery considered to be essential to the specialty: neuroanatomy, neurophysiology, neuropathology, neuroradiology, clinical neurology, general surgery and neurosurgery proper. To provide sufficient test content to assure the reliability of five specified subscores, the examination called for 500 questions and a total time allowance of six hours.

At the outset, the commission had intended to offer the examination to residents completing residency training within two years. It was felt that this would allow adequate time for additional study to correct any areas of weakness disclosed by the examination. Any individual who had already completed his formal training and who wished to take the examination would be allowed to do so, however. In fact, individuals who had previously failed the certifying examination (an entirely oral examination) were encouraged to take the in-training examinations to gain further information about their continuing educational needs.

From the beginning of this program, both the commission and the Board of Neurological Surgery had emphasized that the examination should be regarded as an in-training evaluation for the purposes of identifying weaknesses in a trainee's preparation and in the training program. Throughout the planning and implementation of the study, all concerned held firmly to the view that the individual results should neither be published nor revealed to the Board. A trainee's performance on the in-training examination could not, therefore, be used at a later date to influence his acceptance for the final certifying examination, nor could it be used by the specialty board to influence the decision as to whether he passed or failed the final examination.

Accordingly, it was decided that a trainee's score for the examination as a whole and his subscores on the component categories would be made available only to the chairman of the commission, and through him to the trainee himself and to the director of his training program. Thus, only the trainee and his program director would have the opportunity of discussing the scores.

The first in-training examination in neurosurgery was administered in 1964.

Completely new examinations, but comparable in content, were developed and administered annually thereafter, and residents had the opportunity to take repeat examinations during the period of their training.

No passing level was applied to the examinations. Each examinee received a score report for the total examination and for each of five subtests; each also received frequency distributions in such detail as to permit comparison with others at the same level of training, or at more advanced or less advanced levels, referring to designated subcategories of subject matter. Thus, a candidate might be deficient in neuroradiology but better than average in other categories of the test. Both the candidate and the program director could then take appropriate steps to strengthen the neuroradiology.

As the program proceeded, impartial and reliable data derived from the examinations served to fulfill the primary objectives set forth by the commission: to provide direction for learning, leading to improvement in the competence of candidates for Board certification, and also to provide a means for the objective evaluation of individual training programs. By 1970, the results of the six-year study showed that the Board had achieved its objective leading to better preparation for the oral examination. The written examination was then added to the certification process and the oral examination was modified accordingly.

Other specialty societies have sought the assistance of the National Board in developing examinations for the specific purpose of aiding the learning of the resident. As in the case of Neurological Surgery, the National Board works with committees of the specialty societies responsible for the definition, design and content of the examinations. Subscores are derived in the major subject-matter categories. Scores for individual examinees are obtained for each subcategory and for the examination as a whole. The scores, with frequency distributions based upon levels of training similar to those distributions for the neurosurgery examinations, provide detailed information for the resident to assess his own areas of relative strength or weakness.

Self-assessment for Continuing Medical Education

Multiple-choice testing methods, having gained wide recognition for accurate measurement of medical knowledge, are being applied increasingly to a different and yet closely related phase of medical education usually referred to as continuing medical education.

Traditionally, continuing medical education has been available through assiduous reading of professional journals and through periodic attendance at medical meetings and participation in postgraduate courses offered by medical schools, hospitals and specialty societies. In 1966 a program sponsored by the American Medical Association and known as the Utah Pilot Study undertook to determine, together with other information, the physician's perception of his own educational needs. This information was then to serve as a basis for structuring the content of postgraduate courses.[7,8] A questionnaire was distributed to physicians throughout the state asking them to indicate those areas of medical knowledge in which they felt deficient; in a sense, the physician was asked to specify what he did not know. Obviously the program left much to be desired. If an individual had not even heard of some recent and perhaps important advance in medical knowledge, how could he possibly indicate this in responding to the questionnaire?

A different approach was initiated by the American College of Physicians in 1967.[9,10] The objective was much the same: to provide an opportunity for the physician to identify for himself any gaps in his knowledge so that he could then take steps to educate himself in those areas in which he had found himself deficient. The method, however, was different and far more realistic: It provided the physician with a comprehensive set of multiple-choice test questions which he could study confidentially on his own time, testing his own knowledge of the major areas of internal medicine.

To implement the program, Hugh Butt, formerly chairman of the College's Committee on Educational Activities, requested the National Board to assist in an innovative project that became known as the Medical Knowledge Self-assessment Program. Sets of multiple-choice questions were formulated by nine specially appointed committees of the College. Each committee consisted of about six individuals and was responsible for one of nine major areas of internal medicine: hematology, pulmonary disease, endocrinology and metabolism, renal disease and electrolytes, rheumatology, infectious disease and allergy, gastroenterology, cardiology and neurology. To provide adequate coverage of each of the special areas, approximately 80 multiple-choice questions were agreed upon as the goal for each committee. The total set of questions, therefore, amounted to 720.

The committee members formulated questions according to an outline of subject matter they themselves had devised. They then met with the medical and technical staff of the National Board, at which time the questions were accepted, revised or discarded. Emphasis was placed upon current knowledge and concepts, with special attention to new advances applicable to the practice of medicine.

The author of each question was requested to cite one or more references; these were later assembled as a bibliography and sent to each member participating in the program with a report indicating the questions he had answered correctly and incorrectly. The hope and expectation were that he would study the references for each question he had answered incorrectly, and thus would fill in the gaps in his knowledge.

Here then was a new enterprise applying the experience and technical know-how of designing examinations for precise measurements of individuals and groups to a new mode of continuing medical education. This form of self-assessment and self-learning was soon emulated by other specialty societies; it not only grew rapidly but also led to the development of a widening variety of ways by which to allow the participant to benefit from his experience.

Methods for Developing the Learning Potential of Examinations

Any examination, whether of essay or multiple-choice questions, has the potential of calling to the attention of the examinee the gaps in the knowledge expected by the examiner. These gaps, having been identified, have a potential for informal or formally structured corrective learning. In the National Board examinations for purposes of certification and qualification for license, this potential is not utilized. The policy of the National Board is to hold secure and not to release any multiple-choice questions that have been used in its formal examinations. There are strong reasons for holding strictly to this policy: (1) Performance statistics derived from previously used items serve as the basis for comparison and standardization of examinations from year to year. (2) Reuse of test questions that have not been available for student study and review avoids an horrendous task that would arise in the formulation of completely new tests for each administration (e.g., about 1,000 items for a total Part I). (3) Release of used test items would inevitably lead to review and publication of tests that would be avidly used by students in preparation for a qualifying examination—a rather poor pedagogical exercise.

At the practice level, the situation is quite different. For undergraduate medical education, extramural qualifying examinations are designed as instruments to measure the knowledge and competence of individuals; complications can arise in departure from this objective. At the practice level, however, the objective of self-assessment examinations is to identify gaps in the knowledge of an individual so that these gaps may be corrected.

One approach to this objective was the initial procedure of the American College of Physicians in which, as noted above, the participants in the test received from the College their test answer papers with indications of right and wrong responses together with a list of references for each question, so that they could study those references keyed to the questions answered incorrectly.

The Syllabus

A more comprehensive form of feedback for corrective learning was introduced by the American College of Radiology. This College, also in consultation with ths National Board, developed what became known as their Professional Self-evaluation Continuing Education Program. In the first year of the program, 100 multiple-choice questions, each accompanied by one or more roentgenograms, were written in the field of diseases of the chest. The committee responsible for the test questions also prepared a syllabus containing a brief discussion explaining why the correct response was correct and furthermore why each of the incorrect responses was incorrect.[11] This syllabus was made available after the self-assessment test had been completed and the answer papers returned to the individual participants, who could then make a careful study of the questions in which they had gone wrong. Subsequently, similar programs and syllabi have been published by the American College of Radiology covering the fields of bone disease, genitourinary disease, head and neck disease, pediatrics, nuclear radiology and radiation pathology.

A somewhat different syllabus was that of the American College of Physicians in their third model of their Medical Knowledge Self-assessment Program. (New self-assessment programs have been developed at three-year intervals since the first in 1968.) In this instance, the syllabus was not related to specific questions but dealt more generally with discussion of major topics. It was issued before the self-assessment program with an announcement that an examination for recertification in internal medicine would follow, drawn in part from the self-assessment examination questions. This was powerful inducement indeed for subscription to the self-assessment and for careful study of the syllabus, not only for the self-assessment but more importantly for the recertification examination in internal medicine first administered by the American Board of Internal Medicine in 1974.[12]

Key-word Feedback*

Even when, as noted above, it is considered important to maintain the security of examination questions so that they may be used again for future qualifying examinations, it is still possible to provide the examinee with detailed information about the questions that were answered incorrectly. A technique has been devised using key words to identify the main features of each question. These key words are then coded and keypunched for computer storage. Through simple programming, it is then possible for each examinee to receive a computer-generated printout of key words describing each item that was answered incorrectly on an examination.

An example of this type of feedback is an individualized report of performance on an examination in anesthesiology. The report gave the total score and subscores for the subtests. Percentage scores recorded the percentage of questions answered correctly in that category; the standard scores represented the examinee's relative performance with respect to other examinees. For each question answered incorrectly key-word phrases were listed. Each key-word phrase is a concise description of a concept or fact pertaining to a question on the examination. In the test's subcategory of anatomy, examples of key-word phrases might be: root innervation of hand muscles, shoulder muscles—action, or Horner's syndrome—causes. In the subcategory of physiology, examples might be: EEG—drug effects, brain waves—source, or myotonia—EMG. A typical listing of key-word phrases might cover two pages in the individual examinee's performance report.

Feedback for Patient Management Problems (PMP)

When patient management problems (PMP) were introduced into self-assessment examinations, a different type of feedback was needed. In this type of question, there is no single correct response (see description of PMP, pages 40–47, and sample PMP in Appendix B, pages 170–178). For a learning feedback, it is important that each option be identified as to whether it was considered essential, important, unimportant or dangerous to the management of the patient. Table 1 shows an example of the way in which an examinee, when his scored papers are returned to him, may count up the total number of responses that had been selected in each score category according to the indicated degree of rightness or wrongness. The numbers listed in the column "my count" may then be compared against the "ideal count" demonstrating to the examinee whether the total score indicates overordering, underordering, appropriate selectivity in ordering or even, possibly, the selection of dangerous or life-threatening options.

* This procedure was initiated by The Council of Resident Education in Obstetrics and Gynecology and followed by an increasing number of specialty boards.

Table 1. Scoring Sheet

		Number of Options Selected	
	Types of Options	Ideal Count	My Count
Score	Description		
−5	life-threatening	0	_____
−3	harmful: nonproductive, time consuming, or adds cost	0	_____
−1	not harmful: but nonproductive, time consuming, or adds cost	0	_____
+1	helpful for diagnosis and treatment	8	_____
+3	important for diagnosis and treatment	3	_____
+5	essential for diagnosis and treatment	6	_____

Self-assessment and Evaluation of Self-learning

As noted with reference to state requirements for continuing medical education (see next page), compliance with the requirements was established as depending entirely upon the physician's own report of attendance at scheduled classes, lectures, symposia or "other acceptable educational activities." Objective evaluation of what might have been gained in the educational experience was entirely lacking.

With accumulating experience in the evaluation of learning at all levels of medical education, the National Board of Medical Examiners assisted the College of Physicians of Philadelphia in developing a program that would include assessment of the gain achieved by the individual participant. The National Board contributed its expertise in educational measurement; the College of Physicians of Philadelphia provided the base of an educational institution with one of the foremost medical libraries of the country to serve as a resource for the self-learning.[13] The focus of the program was on the physician in primary medical care—broadly defined as general internal medicine, general pediatrics and family practice. The design of the program included four major steps: (1) an easily completed practice profile to identify the major components of the physician's daily practice,* (2) self-assessment in one or more major areas of the individual's practice, thus identifying in a very personal and detailed way specific learning needs, (3) self-selection of learning materials from the library resources of the College and other sources and (4) a postlearning self-assessment for evaluation of gain and determination of need for further continuing education. The close relationship between the educational features and the practice of the individual physician gave the program its name and its acronym—Practice-related Educational Program (PREP).

To illustrate the general nature of the program, let us assume that following step #1, the practice profile, a physician had learned, perhaps with some

---

* The practice profile devised for this program was a simplified adaptation of a more sophisticated technique developed at the University of Wisconsin and described by Sivertson.[14]

element of surprise, that 60 per cent of his daily practice was in the general field of cardiovascular disease. A self-assessment examination covering this area from the point of view of primary care would then be offered to be done at home. The examination results would indicate in detail that the physician might have become rusty in some aspects and unaware of new advances in other aspects of the major components of his practice as identified in the profile. In the next step, the self-learning phase—which is the central objective of the program—the College provides a list of references from journals or textbooks, audio cassettes, slide cassettes and video cassettes, and may notify the physician of the time and location of lectures or courses in the specified area of learning needs. Thus, the physician-learner's choice of educational opportunities is affected by three components of learning: (1) the subject matter, (2) the time available for learning and (3) perhaps most important, individual preference in method of learning.

Following the learning phase, a self-evaluation of the gain in learning is accomplished by taking a parallel form of the test covering the same health problem area tested at the beginning of the program. Comparisons of the results of the self-assessments before and after the instruction indicate whether or not the learning experiences were effective. The physician can then choose to request more learning materials in the same area, to move to another learning area or to terminate the program.

Two features of PREP were especially attractive to state medical societies and led to its use for purposes of meeting state requirements for continuing medical education. The fact that learning needs were identified in detail in relation to actual practice and materials were made available for corrective study and learning at home base was particularly helpful for the physician at some distance from the opportunities for continuing medical education abundant in major medical centers. Second, the evaluation of the self-learning provided an element of confidence in its effectiveness.

Continuing Medical Education—A Burgeoning Field

Strong incentives have promoted and continue to promote the rapid growth of continuing medical education. An increasing number of state medical societies have adopted policies requiring continuing medical education as a condition of membership. As an even stronger motive, legislation in a growing number of states requires physicians to participate in continuing medical education as a condition for reregistration of the license to practice medicine.

Although relicensure—or more specifically the threat of losing the license to continue to practice one's profession—does indeed sound ominous, the basis of the procedure currently used to meet the requirement softens the threat. The American Medical Association established the Physician's Recognition Award (PRA) which is granted to any physician who gives evidence of having participated in continuing medical education sufficient to acquire 150 credit points during the course of three years. Several categories of credit points were established and published by the American Medical Association.[15] The most important category, Category I, is derived from participation in continuing medical education activities conducted by institutions with accredited sponsorship. Other categories include activities with nonaccredited sponsorship, medical teaching, publication of papers and other "meritorious learning activities."

In the regulations pertaining to the Physician's Recognition Award, the key word is attendance. The physician attends a lecture, course or symposium; he or she receives a certificate specifying the number of credit hours (if the activity qualifies for Category I); this record is then added to others acquired for the needed total of 150. Sometimes the participant is asked for an "evaluation" of the lecture, course or symposium; the accumulated opinions are spoken of as an evaluation. But any element of objective evaluation of the learning gained—or not gained—by the physician is lacking. The question, therefore, arises as to whether the Physician's Recognition Award will continue to be accepted as an adequate indication of continuing competence of the physician for purposes of maintaining membership in a state medical society or renewal of the license to practice.

References

1. Furlow, L. T.: Report of the study commission of the American Board of Neurological Surgery. J. Neurosurg., 27:381, 1967.
2. Hubbard, J. P., Furlow, L. T. and Matson, D. D.: An in-training examination for residents as a guide to learning. N. Engl. J. Med., 276:448, 1967.
3. Levit, E. J.: Comments regarding further study of graduate training in neurosurgery. J. Neurosurg., 27:385, 1967.
4. Levit, E. J.: Evaluation of learning. Arch. Dermatol., 99:343, 1969.
5. Matson, D. D.: An in-training evaluation of residency training programs and trainees. J. Med. Educ., 41:47, 1966.
6. Odom, G. L.: Neurological surgery and the assessment of accomplishment. J. Med. Educ., 44:784, 1969.
7. Castle, C. H. and Storey, P. B.: Physicians' needs and interests in continuing medical education. JAMA, 206:611, 1968.
8. Storey, P. B. and Castle, C. H.: Continuing Medical Education. American Medical Association, Chicago, 1968.
9. Butt, H. R.: Medical knowledge self-assessment program. Bull. Am. Coll. Physicians, September 1967.
10. Rosenow, E. C., Jr.: The medical knowledge self-assessment program, J. Med. Educ., 44:706, 1969.
11. Chest Disease Syllabus. American College of Radiology, Chicago, 1972.
12. Medical Knowledge Self-assessment Program IV. Syllabus 1977. American College of Physicians, Philadelphia, 1977.
13. Bowles, F. L., Brading, P. L., Burg, F. D., Finestone, A. J. and Hubbard, J. P.: A practice-related education program. JAMA, 237:1346, 1977.
14. Sivertson, S. E., et al.: Initial physician profile: Continuing education related to medical practice. J. Med. Educ., 48:1006, 1973.
15. Medical Education in the United States. 76th Annual Report. JAMA, 236:2949, 1976.

CHAPTER 10

■

Research and Development
Barbara J. Andrew

As reflected in its bylaws, the National Board of Medical Examiners regards research and development as major responsibilities. Collectively, the Board's research and development efforts have emerged from a conviction that the precision of existing assessment procedures can be continuously enhanced and that new technology combined with imagination and insight can produce innovations that will in fact enhance the evaluation of professional competence. In order to be prepared to respond appropriately to requests for new evaluation services, research and development studies are also conducted to anticipate the impact that emerging trends may have on the evaluation of health professionals. Finally, research and development are compelling activities of the Board because of their inherent intellectual attraction and because of the Board's awareness of its public and professional accountability for the quality of its assessment procedures.

The National Board's mission lies in the development of measurement techniques and evaluation methodologies that can be used to evaluate (1) individual competence in the health professions and (2) the effectiveness of policies and programs in health education and health care delivery.

Activities encompassed in this overall mission include the development of instrumentation and appropriate scoring strategies, studies of the validity and reliability of these instruments and investigations of the economic and logistic feasibility of implementing them on a local and national scale. Studies also focus on the extent to which assessment capability has been enhanced by the introduction of new methodologies and on the extent to which clusters of instruments yield more potent assessments than any one of them alone. Before instruments can be applied to the real world of evaluation, they must be examined to analyze what they can and cannot assess, how they can be best utilized, what their cost-effectiveness is and how the resulting data can be used appropriately for decision making. Moreover, decision makers must be aware of the different interpretations that can be drawn from data, depending upon the statistical and analytical procedures applied to them.

Because of the complexity of the National Board's mission in research and development, it is regarded as an institutional activity. Although the Research and Development Department provides leadership and the focus of staff expertise, the conceptualization and implementation of individual research and development projects are carried out by project teams that represent an appropriate interdepartmental mix of staff resources. In order to provide an environment capable of supporting and nurturing individual creativity and initiative and enriching these through constructive critical review and collaboration among colleagues and peers, the work of the project teams is guided by two groups: the Staff Research Committee and the project advisory committees. The Staff Research Committee provides interdepartmental review of research proposals and reports, while the project advisory committees consist of external consultants appointed to develop evaluation materials for specific projects and to advise project teams about content and methodological issues. The Advisory Committee on Research and Development, which played a major role in establishing the Research and Development Department, provides policy advice to the National Board with respect to its overall plan for research and development and the identification of research priorities. The Advisory Committee also reviews and approves research proposals and provides guidance in funding strategies.

Historically, the financial resources for research and development at the National Board have come primarily from private foundations. Since the early 1970s, the Board has invested an increasing amount of its own financial resources in research and development and has relied as well upon grants and contracts from federal agencies to provide a major share of the support for these efforts. The number of projects cosponsored with medical specialty boards has also grown. These organizations not only provide partial financial support for projects but contribute board members to project advisory committees and serve as sources of contact for the recruitment of participants for field trials.

Historical Overview

Research and development at the National Board began in 1951 when the Educational Testing Service was asked to help the Board develop multiple-choice tests and assess their effectiveness in relation to the essay examinations which were then used for physician licensure. At that time, the National Board did not have a professional psychometric staff and thus, as noted in Chapter 1, the collaborative arrangement with a larger, more experienced testing firm was necessary. Although the American Board of Internal Medicine had already converted its certifying examination from essay to multiple-choice format, the conversion of National Board tests was viewed with suspicion, and regarded by some within the professional community as an anti-intellectual trend which would be likely to dilute the quality of the evaluation of professional competence.[1] During the initial period of study,* comparisons were made of the relationships between performance on multiple-choice and essay tests and medical school grades. For the two subtests on which the comparisons were made (medicine and pharmacology), stronger positive relationships were observed for the multiple-choice questions than for the essay questions (.37, .49 vs. .21, .18).[2] Subsequent studies of the other Part I and Part II subtests provided sufficient statistical support for the new objective test questions to result in a

---

* This work was supported by the Markle Foundation.

conversion of the entire Part I and Part II examinations from essay to multiple-choice questions.[3] The effects of this decision were not altogether realized at first, but in due course it significantly altered the nature of testing for medical licensure and influenced the testing procedures used by most medical schools. In addition, the National Board's internal test development procedures were converted to the test committee method, which provided for the development and review of test questions by a group of experts rather than by a single examiner.

During this period of change in Parts I and II, the Part III examination continued as an oral and bedside evaluation of "clinical competence." As the number of candidates to be tested began to increase rapidly, numerous problems affecting the logistics and feasibility of test administration were encountered. Of even greater importance, however, was a growing concern among staff, test committees and the Board about the extent to which the oral and bedside examinations were really assessing important elements of clinical competence. As a result, in 1958 a grant was obtained from the Rockefeller Foundation and the American Institutes for Research (AIR) was asked to conduct a two-year empirical study to identify important components of clinical competence. By means of a critical incident technique, over 3,300 instances of good and poor physician behavior were collected from clinical faculty who had observed the performance of interns and residents. These incidents were analyzed and classified into nine major categories of clinical competence, with suggestions for approaches to the evaluation of each.[4]

In order to incorporate the findings of this critical incident study into the development of innovative testing procedures, the National Board staff undertook an extensive analysis of the competency components documented in the final report. As a result, motion picture film examinations and patient management problems (see Chapter 4) were introduced into Part III in 1961. Patient photographs, roentgenograms and other clinical data presented in pictorial and graphic format were also introduced with accompanying multiple-choice questions.[5] These new testing procedures dramatically changed the content and format of the Part III examination, and the demonstrated feasibility of printing pictorial materials in test booklets influenced specialty boards in eliminating their traditional "slide quiz"—the projection of slide materials during the written examination.

The AIR critical incident study, which resulted in the development of these major innovations in testing methodology, also led to the introduction of a more objective approach to the bedside examination which continued to be included as a component of Part III until 1964. By that time, the results of a three-year empirical study had demonstrated the reliability of the new testing methodologies, and additional studies had revealed the unreliability of observations made during the bedside examination. This statistical evidence, along with increasing costs and logistic difficulties, resulted in elimination of the bedside examination and expanded utilization of the innovative testing procedures noted above.

During the period in which the Part III examination was undergoing these major revisions, the Part II test committees expressed interest in undertaking a critical review of the content and format of their examination. As a result of this study (supported by the Commonwealth Fund), refinements were made in the content outlines from which test questions were developed. Pictorial and graphic materials were introduced in relation to multiple-choice questions and were used for the first time as response alternatives rather than as accompaniments to the introductory stems of test questions. In addition, analysis of the test materials submitted by the test committees suggested considerable overlap of testing content across the clinical specialties. As a result of this finding, separate subject scores continued to be derived for reporting purposes but were no longer used as separate hurdles for determining pass/fail. Thereafter, pass/fail decisions were based on a composite score. (A similar change in the scoring of Part I was made several years later.)

Once the content and format of the Part I, II, and III examinations had become reasonably stable, a series of validation studies was conducted during the last half of the 1960s. For Parts I and II, these studies consisted of correlational analyses between performance on the examinations and medical school grades. Significant positive relationships (ranging from .31 to .86) were consistently found between these variables.[6] For the Part III examination, validation studies (funded by grants from The Commonwealth Fund and the Carnegie Corporation) consisted of comparisons between the performance of third-year medical students and interns in order to determine whether expected differences in the clinical competence of these groups would be reflected in their examination scores. Such differences were found in the analyses of data.[7] In addition, at the request of the military services, the Part III examination was administered at the beginning and end of the internship year in all Army, Navy and Air Force hospitals over a three-year period. Significant gains in performance were found by the end of the internship year, and, in addition, significant positive relationships (.39 and .47) were found between performance on the Part III examination and faculty and peer ratings of clinical performance.[8]

In 1968, a portion of the grant support provided by the Carnegie Corporation, as noted above, was used to conduct a study of the relevance of Parts I and II. A special task force was appointed to review and select previously used test materials to be included in the study. With the cooperation of 108 medical school faculties throughout the United States and Canada, an attempt was made to probe faculty opinion regarding the extent to which National Board examination questions were assessing knowledge and skills compatible with the objectives of the medical school curricula.[9] In general, faculty opinion supported the relevance of the content of the two examinations. In addition, this work, in part, provided impetus for the introduction of testing in the behavioral sciences.

By 1968, the National Board's experience with patient management problems and the staff's awareness of rapidly expanding computer technology and studies of individualized testing led to a decision to investigate the use of computer-simulation techniques in assessing complex cognitive skills in clinical medicine. Preliminary discussions were held with the staff at the Laboratory for Computer Sciences of the Massachusetts General Hospital and the Department of Continuing Education at Harvard Medical School. As a result of these discussions, a joint effort combining expertise in testing and measurement with expertise in designing computerized diagnostic simulations was undertaken. With funding from The Commonwealth Fund and the Carnegie Corporation, a prototype computer-based examination was designed to assess judgment in selecting and interpreting diagnostic data from the history, physical examination and laboratory studies.[10] Its successful demonstration at the 1970 meeting of the American College of Physicians reflected considerable receptivity to the new technology and enthusiasm within the profession for this method of evaluating skills in medical diagnosis.

Recent Studies

Based upon the success of the prototype computer-based examination (CBX), a three-year joint research program was undertaken in 1971 by the National Board of Medical Examiners and the American Board of Internal Medicine. Additional grants were received from the Carnegie Corporation and The Commonwealth Fund to continue development of a computer-based system for assessing clinical competence and to address validation and networking issues.[11] Findings from the first phase of national field trials showed limited but promising differences in the performance of groups of physicians with hypothesized differences in clinical competence. The study of networking problems concluded that national computer testing was within the realm of possibility, and a comparative study of several scoring strategies provided valuable information regarding useful approaches in evaluating physician performance on the simulated cases.[12] Because it was felt that the observed differences in performance could be further highlighted by modifying the simulation model to focus more heavily on the clinical judgment associated with patient management and treatment strategies, a second phase of research and development was conceptualized.

This second phase of work on CBX is directed by a project staff at the University of Wisconsin School of Medicine at Madison and funded principally by grants from the Robert Wood Johnson Foundation and the Charles E. Merrill Trust. The two sponsoring Boards and the University of Wisconsin also provided financial support for the project. The effectiveness of the new simulation model is to be evaluated by comparing physician performance on the simulated cases with performance in actual practice as assessed by a review of medical records. In addition, performances on the simulated cases by residents in internal medicine are being compared with ratings of their clinical performance. Evaluation parameters in the new model include outcome measures such as the cost, risk and complication rates of management and therapy decisions. Studies of new scoring strategies and current networking alternatives are also being conducted.

In 1972, as a result of the deliberations of the Board's Committee on Goals and Priorities,[13] a decision was reached to develop an evaluation program for the certification of assistants to the primary care physician.* This program marked the National Board's first departure from the assessment of the competence of physicians, but seemed compatible with its mission because of the functions of physician's assistants and their relationship to practicing physicians. In addition to the development of a written examination, several validation and research studies were undertaken.

---

* This project was funded by the Robert Wood Johnson Foundation, the W. K. Kellogg Foundation and the Department of Health, Education and Welfare.

The validation studies disclosed significant differences in performance between students at the beginning and end of formal training, and significant positive relationships between examination performance and ratings of clinical competence.[14,15]

A research study was also undertaken to develop behavioral checklists to assess techniques in performing a physical examination of the major body systems.[16] Field studies of this technique demonstrated reasonably high reliabilities among observers and significant differences in performance between groups of physician's assistants with hypothesized differences in physical examination skills. As a result, this aspect of performance testing was introduced as part of the overall examination program.

Because of the growing interest in criterion-referenced procedures for setting examination standards, several such procedures were studied.[17] It was found that different approaches resulted in significantly different examination standards, and the same criterion-referenced approach used by different groups of judges also resulted in significantly different standards. Because of these findings the pass/fail level for the certifying examination continued to be based upon the traditional norm-referenced procedures. During the same period, a parallel study was conducted by the American Board of Pediatrics with assistance from the National Board staff, and similar conclusions were reached.

In 1972, a collaborative project between the National Board, the R.S. McLaughlin Examination and Research Centre at the University of Alberta, Canada, and the American Board of Pediatrics was conducted to assess the effect of computerizing patient management problems written for the paper-and-pencil format. One objective of the study was to determine whether the availability of visual access to later sections of a patient management problem had any effect on performance in the early sections. Such visual access was not possible with the computerized PMPs. The study found significant differences between performance on the paper-and-pencil and the computerized patient management problems (confirming the hypothesis that visual access had an effect upon scores).[18] However, the study also found that the reliability and validity of the patient-management problems under study were essentially the same for the paper-and-pencil version as for the computerized version. Although the computerized PMPs were well received by the examinees who participated in the study, the associated costs discouraged implementation of this methodology.

Until the early 1970s, the National Board's research and development efforts focused on the conceptualization and field study of indirect testing methods for assessing individual competence. By 1971, the manner in which medical records were being used to evaluate institutional performance patterns and quality of care prompted the National Board staff to become interested in the potential use of medical record audits to assess certain aspects of individual physician performance. Although this early staff interest preceded activities of the Professional Standards Review Organization and policies regarding the periodic recertification of physician competence, these subsequent trends only heightened our conviction that new methodologies were needed to provide more direct assessments of actual physician performance.

Accordingly, in 1973 a collaborative project was undertaken by the National Board of Medical Examiners and the American Board of Pediatrics to investigate the utilization of medical record audits in ambulatory care settings.* The study was designed: (1) to assess the feasibility of instituting medical record audits of resident performance, (2) to investigate the number of observations required to obtain a stable estimate of physician performance and (3) to evaluate the relationship between compliance with audit criteria and performance on a written in-training examination. The latter evaluation would, it was hoped, provide an estimate of the extent to which these two methodologies were assessing overlapping dimensions of competence. Audit criteria were developed for seven pediatric medical conditions; record auditors were recruited and trained, and five institutions participated in the study.[19]

The data from this study indicated that reasonably reliable estimates of physician performance could be obtained with a sample of ten records in a given medical problem area. When reliability was assessed using a measure of internal consistency, reliability coefficients ranged from .49 to .90. These reliability estimates were affected by the number of criteria specified for each medical condition, so that reliability increased as the number of criteria increased. The estimates of relationship between performance on the in-training examination and compliance with audit criteria suggested that there was very little overlap between the two evaluation methodologies and that performance as assessed by one methodology could not be used as a predictor of performance on the other.[20]

In 1975, the National Board received a request to participate in a medical record self-audit project sponsored by the National Heart, Lung, and Blood Institute. This presented an opportunity to expand the National Board's experience with record audits and to evaluate the effectiveness of physicians' use of their own medical records as a self-assessment technique. Criteria for the initial and follow-up evaluations of hypertensive patients were developed by two committees, one focusing on care in an institutional setting and the other on care in an office practice. These two sets of criteria along with the self-audit materials are being field tested in several hospital locations and then in office practices.[21]

In yet another application of medical record audits to evaluation purposes, the National Board responded to a request by the Department of Health, Education, and Welfare to conduct a validation study of the Physician's Assistant Certifying Examination using an audit of office medical records as the criterion measure of performance. One hundred sixteen physician's assistants who had taken the 1974 Certifying Examination volunteered to participate in this study. Audit criteria were developed for twelve medical conditions, and a group of seven medical record administrators and technicians were trained in using these criteria to audit office records. The resulting data did not show any consistent pattern of significant relationships between examination performance and compliance with audit criteria. Moreover, a number of logistic and measurement problems associated with conducting record audits were highlighted for further study.[14]

Until the early 1970s, the major testing interest of the National Board focused on the assessment of knowledge and related cognitive skills. However, the observation was inescapable that the components of clinical competence

* This work was supported by the Department of Health, Education and Welfare and the participating Boards.

identified by the AIR critical incident study extended into other areas of behavior, including interpersonal and communication skills. Thus, the scope of competency components for which the National Board was to conduct research was expanded.

One of the principal challenges facing the Board was to develop a comprehensive definition of interpersonal skills and to define performance criteria. The feasibility of achieving these objectives was doubted by many who felt that interpersonal skills constituted a "soft" area of evaluation.

A review of the literature suggested that investigators at various medical schools were making headway in defining interpersonal skills and in developing observation systems for assessing physician-patient interaction. The National Board undertook two research efforts, one focusing on the assessment of interpersonal skills of physicians and the other on the assessment of interpersonal skills of physician's assistants. Both projects began with the difficult question of definitions. A group consensus approach was used to develop behavioral statements describing good and poor interpersonal skills. The earlier AIR critical incident study and definitions developed by other investigators served as the basis for the initial work in defining this competency component.

The Physician Interpersonal Skills Project team designed a nonevaluative system for observing behavioral patterns during a physician-patient interaction. Observers who were not physicians were trained to view videotaped interactions and to code at three-second intervals the behaviors they observed. A two-dimensional matrix was designed so that the patterns of interaction could be displayed graphically. Other approaches to the evaluation of live interaction were also designed, including ratings provided by simulated patients, medical students and physicians. These evaluation formats will be compared one with another, with specified outcome measures, and with case write-ups provided by each medical student following the patient interview. Finally, the interaction analysis system will be used as the criterion measure in evaluating the effectiveness of multiple-choice questions with and without videotape accompaniment as indirect measures of interpersonal skills.

The initial period of this investigation was funded by an award from the W.T. Grant Foundation. In 1976, the American Board of Family Practice became a cosponsor of the project and has provided financial support along with the National Board of Medical Examiners. In 1977, the Josiah Macy Jr. Foundation provided additional support as part of a collaborative effort of the National Board, the Educational Testing Service and a consortium of 13 medical schools.

The project designed to assess the interpersonal skills of physician's assistants also began with the development of a mechanism for observing and recording interaction during the patient interview. The primary focus of this project, however, was the development of an interactive audiovisual simulation system which could be used to simulate a patient interview using branching videotape scripts. The system was designed to attempt to capture the branching, interactive and audiovisual dimensions of the patient interviewing process. Branching paper-and-pencil simulations and problem-centered multiple-choice questions were also developed with the objective of comparing the magnitude of correlation between performance on these three simulation techniques and interviewing performance as measured by audio recordings of live interviews. Analyses of preliminary field trials disclosed modest relationships (.39 to .42) between audio recordings of live interviews and performance on the paper-and-pencil simulations and audiovisual simulations with respect to one of three variables studied (patient-oriented inquiries). No significant relationships were observed when performance was assessed by multiple-choice questions.*[22]

Force Fields and Trends

Throughout its history, the National Board's research has focused principally on the development of evaluation methodologies for the assessment of the competence of the physician. Following the introduction of objective testing made possible by the multiple-choice technique, other innovations conceived by the National Board were motion pictures and photographs depicting clinical findings, patient management problems, a prototype computer-based examination, an interactive audiovisual simulation system and an interaction analysis system for documenting physician-patient behavioral patterns. Three common threads have linked National Board research efforts to date: (1) the development of more comprehensive and detailed definitions of the components of clinical competence, (2) the assessment of individual performance (rather than that of groups, systems, or institutions) and (3) the attainment of increased objectivity and standardization of the evaluation process.

In most instances, research has led to the development of new methods or refinements in existing techniques. However, evaluation procedures such as the bedside and oral examinations have been discontinued when empirical investigations demonstrated they could not meet acceptable standards of reliability and objectivity. Lest it be thought that the National Board has been ruled by statistics alone, it should be pointed out that major decisions have at all times and at all stages in the development of new procedures been influenced by the critical judgments of the members of the National Board and especially its project advisory committee members and examiners (see Chapter 2) who, as has been noted, are recognized experts in their fields.

While there have been no failures as such, some research studies have resulted in the decision not to adopt a procedure for operational purposes. As an example, several criterion-referenced standard-setting procedures were studied, and the findings did not warrant a substitution of these newer procedures for the traditional norm-referenced approaches. However, continuing uneasiness with current methods of setting examination standards has prompted the planning of additional studies using different procedures. The introduction of standardized objective testing in the early 1950s produced a strong trend away from the assessment of observed clinical behavior. While the advantages and contributions of objective testing are well recognized, a growing awareness of its limitations has emerged in the last few years, and

* This work is being supported in part by the Department of Health, Education and Welfare.

there has been renewed interest in the direct assessment of performance. The development of behavioral checklists and medical record audits attest to this interest and to the feasibility of using these techniques for purposes of obtaining reliable measurements of clinical competence.

Three forces have had a major influence in shaping research and development at the National Board. Internal forces have stemmed from the concerns of Board committees and staff about the extent to which existing methodologies were accurately assessing the components of competence they were purporting to assess and about the components of competence for which methodologies had not yet been developed and tested. Criticisms of formalized testing procedures which have been levied by faculty and students within the medical education community have also constituted forces which have shaped research at the National Board. These challenges to testing have come through both informal and formal channels, and because of their constructive contribution highlight the need to encourage regular staff interaction with constituents at both the undergraduate and graduate levels of education.

In addition, the expanding network of external social and economic forces is influencing the health professions directly and has indirect implications for the National Board. Concomitant with the increasing accountability of the medical profession to the public has been a mounting concern for accountability of the assessment procedures which are used to evaluate individual competence and the quality of health care. Many of the procedures currently under development have been made feasible by technological advances and are responses to the fully recognized fact that knowledge is a necessary but not sufficient indicator of professional competence. The complex challenges implicit in the evaluation of continuing competence are just beginning to be addressed. The attitudes and personal qualities of health professionals—likely to be important determinants of behavior—have only begun to be investigated, although they are clearly becoming issues of public concern since they are viewed by many as important determinants of the quality and economics of health care delivery.

Furthermore, public concerns regarding competence, ethics and costs will probably have significant impact not only on the nature of health care delivery systems but on the role of individual physicians and other health professionals within these systems. To the extent that the physician's role evolves toward that of a manager of health care services, evaluation of his competence in this area will need to be undertaken. The challenge which faces the National Board is to anticipate the directions of these trends and their potential impact so that the needed assessment strategies can be developed and tested in advance of the immediate need for their implementation.

Organizational and economic decisions in the health care field should not be so narrowly conceived or financially motivated that they adversely affect the quality of care being provided. To avert this possibility, more sophisticated methodologies than those presently available will need to be designed so that competence and quality-of-care issues can be brought more sharply and accurately into focus. The quality of decision making in the future will be in large measure determined by the quality of the data being generated regarding the performance of individuals, units and systems within the health field.

References

1. Watson, C. J.: Some activities and impacts of the American Board of Internal Medicine. JAMA, 138:257, 1948.
2. Cowles, J. T. and Hubbard, J. P.: A comparative study of essay and objective examinations for medical students. J. Med. Educ., 27(Part 2):14, 1952.
3. Cowles, J. T. and Hubbard, J. P.: Validity and reliability of the new objective tests. J. Med. Educ., 29(6):30, 1954.
4. American Institutes for Research: The definition of clinical competence in medicine: Performance dimensions and rationales for clinical skill areas. Palo Alto, California. Reissued May 1976.
5. Hubbard, J. P., Levit, E. J., Schumacher, C. F. and Schnabel, T. G.: An objective evaluation of clinical competence. N. Engl. J. Med., 272:1321, 1965.
6. Schumacher, C. F. and Kelley, P. R., Jr.: Correlation between medical school grades and National Board examination scores: A follow-up report. Unpublished report.
7. Schumacher, C. F.: Validation of the National Board Part III examination against an operationally defined criterion of clinical competence. Unpublished report.
8. Kelley, P. R., Jr., Stumpe, A. R. and Levit, E. J.: A four-year study of the internship in United States Air Force hospitals: an objective measurement of gain in clinical competence. Milit. Med., 135:537, 1970.
9. Kennedy, W. B., Kelley, P. R. and Hubbard, J. P.: The relevance of National Board Part I examinations to medical school curricula: report to medical schools. Unpublished report.
10. Hubbard, J. P., Levit, E. J., Barnett, G. O., Goldfinger, S. E., Dineen, J. J., Farquhar, B. B. and Schumacher, C. F.: Computer-based evaluation of clinical competence. Bull. Am. Coll. Physicians, October 1970.
11. Senior, J. R.: *Toward the Measurement of Competence in Medicine.* National Board of Medical Examiners, Philadelphia, 1976.
12. Schumacher, C. F.: A comparative study of four methods for scoring an experimental computer-based examination for clinical problem solving. Proceedings of the Thirtieth Annual Conference on Research in Medical Education. Association of American Medical Colleges, Chicago, 1974.
13. Evaluation in the Continuum of Medical Education. Report of the Committee on Goals and Priorities of the National Board of Medical Examiners (Mayer, W., Chairman). National Board of Medical Examiners, Philadelphia, 1973.
14. Andrew, B. J., Dowaliby, F. J. and Erviti, V. F.: National program for the evaluation of primary care physician's assistants. Final report. Submitted to the Department of Health, Education and Welfare, July 1976.
15. Dowaliby, F. J. and Andrew, B. J.: Relationship between clinical competence ratings and examination performance. J. Med Educ., 51:181, 1976.
16. Andrew, B. J.: The use of behavioral checklists to evaluate physical examination skills. J. Med. Educ., 52:589, 1977.
17. Andrew, B. J. and Hecht, J.: A preliminary investigation of two procedures for setting examination standards. Educ. Psychol. Meas., 36:45, 1976.
18. Schumacher, C. F., Burg, F. D. and Taylor, C.: Computerization of a patient management problem examination to prevent "retracing." Br. J. Med. Educ., 9:4, 1975.
19. Templeton, B., Erviti, V. F., Bunce, J. V. and Burg, F. D.: Training medical record abstractors to assure high inter-rater reliability. Proceedings of the Fifteenth Annual Conference on Research in Medical Education. Association of American Medical Colleges, San Francisco, 1976.
20. Templeton, B., Erviti, V. F., Bunce, J. V. and Burg, F. D.: Medical audit of pediatric resident performance. Final report. Submitted to the Department of Health, Education and Welfare, 1977.
21. Erviti, V. F., Templeton, B. and Gold, R. A.: Hypertension medical audit study phase I: A field trial in ambulatory care clinics. Presented at the National Conference on High Blood Pressure Control, Washington, April 1977.
22. Andrew, B. J.: The use of structured simulations in assessing interpersonal skills. In preparation.

CHAPTER 11

■

The National Board and the Public Interest: Pertinent Areas of Activity
Robert A. Chase

In the keynote address for the Annual Conference of the National Board of Medical Examiners in 1972, Dr. Rosemary Stevens perceptively noted the developmental phases which have brought the Board to its present position.[1] She pointed out that the National Board of Medical Examiners originated in response to a need—perceived by notable visionaries in medicine—for standardization of procedures for licensure. This first phase of the development of standardization was followed in succession by a phase of specialization, a phase of testing techniques and, currently, a phase of public interest. Continuing progress has been made in each of these four areas since Dr. Stevens' address five years ago, and it seems fitting to note that progress and to cite the role of the National Board of Medical Examiners in the advances in medical evaluation in the public interest.

Standardization in licensure was essentially nonexistent in the first decade of the twentieth century (see Chapter 1). In this era the physician was accountable only to himself. The founding of the Federation of State Medical Boards in 1913 and of the National Board of Medical Examiners in 1915 were significant steps toward more uniform standards for licensure in the various states. The emergence in 1968 of the Federation Licensing Examination (FLEX) (see Chapter 8) was a landmark decision on the part of the Federation of State Medical Boards. The perseverance of the Federation of State Medical Boards, which resulted in the permeation of recognition of the high quality of FLEX, has led to progressive adoption of the FLEX examination by the states until in 1976 all fifty states accepted FLEX (with a standard passing score of 75) as an acceptable demonstration of competence for licensure. The other route to licensure, no less standard than FLEX, is certification by the National Board. Thus the primary objective for which the National Board was founded has been achieved by the cooperative effort of state boards, the Federation of State Medical Boards and the National Board. The national standard which has resulted is at least an assurance to the public against physician incompetence if that incompetence is based on a serious deficiency of knowledge and problem-solving skills. Important to physicians is the easier mobility which results from common standards among states.

During the age of developing specialization, which started significantly in the early part of this century, the National Board was drawn upon for consultation and service. As specialization became more organized and specialists began to assemble with like specialists for intellectual interchange, certification of specialists by education and individual evaluation inevitably emerged. The National Board has played a significant part by aiding specialty boards in their quest for valid and reliable examinations. At present (1977) the National Board of Medical Examiners serves 16 of 22 primary specialty boards.

Indirectly, through the participation of individual members of the Board and its staff, the National Board has contributed to the development of the new hierarchy in medical education, namely, the Coordinating Council on Medical Education and its Liaison Committees. The National Board serves as an Associate Member of the American Board of Medical Specialties, and in this capacity has supported the increasing role of that organization in specialty certification in America. Important decisions, based on the best manpower data available, are dependent upon the interlinkages of these important groups. Although the National Board in its test development activities is responsive at the graduate level, it also expresses opinions on all health professions evaluation through its membership in the various national medical organizations. Both staff members and members of the Board participate in essentially every national organization involved in health professions education.

The age of testing techniques cited by Dr. Stevens got seriously under way in the 1950s (see Chapter 1). It has no termination point, and remains a primary role of the National Board of Medical Examiners. The transition from essay to multiple-choice question tests, the development of patient management problem strategies, new scoring and analysis measures and the use of visual materials exemplify implementation of developed techniques in the age of the science of educational measurement. The entire research effort at present is aimed at continuing development of new strategies to measure components of general competency that have not been subject to objective measurement. For example, interpersonal and motor skills cannot presently be measured objectively by existing methods. Use of simulators, computer interactive examinations, behavioral checklists and audits are examples of new technology currently under study (see Chapter 10).

Although Dr. Stevens considered its phase of public interest to be last in sequence, the age of public interest for the National Board of Medical Examiners started at its birth. More recently, the Board has assertively responded to public issues both in its own right and through its linkage organizations. It is this new thrust that is addressed here.

Validation Strategies

Elsewhere in this volume (Chapter 6) the strategies for examination validation used to meet public accountability are described in detail. As the principal testing organization in medicine, the National Board of Medical Examiners has always felt a sense of responsibility to produce or to help to produce instruments to measure individual competencies reliably and in a valid manner. As the Board has extended its services to various organizations with licensure and certifying authority and responsibility, it has recognized its obligation to encourage these organizations to validate their own evaluation systems. The staff of the National Board of Medical Examiners is helping its several clients in the field of evaluation to mount validation programs to meet that responsibility. When validation is mandated by statute or by public agencies, the National Board has analyzed the regulations for appropriateness in relationship to medical licensing and certifying examinations. For example, when in 1976 the Equal Employment Opportunities Commission guidelines were studied by an interagency Equal Employment Opportunity Coordinating Council (EEOCC), several changes were recommended, including the proposal that the EEOC guidelines should apply to licensing and certifying organizations in the professions. The National Board's staff, as a matter of public interest, analyzed the guidelines and developed a lengthy critique which was forwarded to EEOCC and to the medical organizations affected. The Board's commentary formed a base document for many organizational responses from medicine's private sector. It is of course essential for the National Board of Medical Examiners and other medical licensing and certifying organizations to validate their evaluation methods. However, the validation process itself must not be such as to threaten the rigor of the test instruments. Some excerpts from the critique to EEOCC may serve as examples of the Board's thrust in response to the EEOC guidelines.

To every extent possible, evaluation methods in medical certification must be free of racial, ethnic or sexual bias, but at the same time they must discriminate adequately regarding the competence of applicants to serve the public as professionals. In principle one must not let what it perceived as adverse impact on employment opportunities of minority or any other groups to become, in fact, adverse impact on the assurance of the quality of medical professionals for the protection of the public.

Because medical certifying examinations, and to an important extent medical licensure examinations, are more a part of the continuum of medical education than they are absolutely discriminatory entrance evaluations, it is inappropriate that they be considered in the same manner as are general employee selection procedures under the guidelines.

There are competencies in decision making, knowledge, clinical skills, and problem-solving abilities that are measurable and are relevant and essential in the documentation of the professional competencies of physicians for their certification and licensure. Evaluations of these competencies are justly and appropriately to be used to protect the public against incompetent medical practice.

It is urged that it be recognized that the guidelines do not give appropriate and adequate consideration to the special problems that arise in evaluation of the complex competencies of medical professionals for the service and protection of the public interest.

Conclusion—The agencies responsible for medical professional evaluation, certification, and licensure have long been involved in developing and maintaining the highest standards of objectivity, reliability and validity of certifying examinations. Their improvement continues to be a goal of the highest priority for these agencies.

There is, however, concern that an attempt to meet forms of validation in the guidelines as proposed would erode the present high standards of evaluation for licensure and certification in medicine and would inhibit further efforts to assure the quality of health care available for the public.

For these sound reasons, certification and licensure in professional areas such as the practice of medicine should not be included within the proposed guidelines.

As for the National Board examinations themselves, there is a substantial history of examination validation study in terms of content, criterion and construct validation, as described in Chapter 6.

Above and beyond the validity of test instruments per se according to acceptable educational psychology principles is the matter of examination security and integrity. As National Board examination test questions have become more and more important as determinants for graduation, licensure and immigration, pressures to gain advance access to such material have grown. Special commercial cram courses to help individuals to prepare for examinations of all sorts have flourished. The National Board has felt a strong obligation to protect the integrity of its examination material both before and during its use (see Chapter 5). The obvious intent is to protect the public against health professionals whose credentials are acquired in a felonious manner.

Educational Continuum

Through serial endorsement and implementation of some recommendations made by the Committee on Goals and Priorities,[2] the Board is taking initiatives to support medical education as a continuum. By this support the National Board of Medical Examiners is catalyzing the implementation of general recommendations to the profession and public made in such notable reports as: (1) Coggeshall Report—Planning for Medical Progress through Education—1965, (2) Millis Report—Graduate Education of Physicians—1966,[3] (3) Carnegie Commission Report—Higher Education and the Nation's Health—1970[4] and (4) HEW—Proposal for Credentialing Health Manpower—1976.[5]

One of the initiatives being taken by the National Board of Medical Examiners in relationship to the recommendations of the Committee on Goals and Priorities is the development of a comprehensive examination specifically designed to evaluate a graduating M.D.'s readiness to assume responsibility for patient care at the level expected in a graduate residency. This is a response to the firm statement endorsed by the Association of American Medical Colleges and American Medical Association that a physician, at the time he acquires his M.D. degree, is not equipped to enter independent medical practice. Thus he is not eligible, nor should he be, for full licensure for independent practice. Nonetheless, the new M.D. assumes a level of patient care within a residency at this critical time. It seems sensible therefore that the public be assured of his demonstrated capability to assume such responsibility. The National Board, anticipating that the appropriate responsible agency may require such an evaluation, undertook in 1975 to prepare a prototype examination and the development of methods for measuring more broadly the competencies required for patient care responsibility at the residency level. The new examination, called the Comprehensive Qualifying Examination (CQE), under development in the late 1970s, I would predict will be in use in the early 1980s.

Response to HEW Need

A sudden need for an examination comparable to the CQE arose with the passage of the Health Professions Education Assistance Act of 1976 (PL 94–484) in October 1976 (see pages 83,84). The National Board responded by the development of a Visa Qualifying Examination (VQE) which served the need by being equivalent to Part I and Part II for the purposes of the law as Congress had intended (see Chapter 8). This action by the National Board of Medical Examiners is an example of its responsive and responsible action in the public interest.

The Department of HEW during the years 1971 to 1977 was evolving a policy toward licensure and certification of health care personnel. The first HEW document, a Report on Licensure and Related Health Personnel Credentialing, appeared in 1971. It was followed by a number of other documents on this subject but all dealt primarily with allied health personnel. In 1976, a publication was produced for review and public discussion to help crystallize HEW policy. The document, A Proposal for Credentialing Health Manpower (June 1976), explicitly applied to "the entire range of health manpower categories" including physicians.[5]

Following careful study and analysis, the National Board staff developed a lengthy response to the monograph, composed of comments about each of the six major recommendations. Since many of the proposed recommendations had to do with evaluation procedures, standards for licensure and certification and national examinations to promote interstate equivalency, the expertise of the Board's staff was essential to develop a proper response from the private sector of medicine. The Board's analysis of the proposal was used in part or in whole by a number of prestigious national organizations in medicine in their own responses to the HEW pamphlet. Many of the recommendations made good sense in terms of public interest but others required thoughtful revision lest they result in establishment of policy that would be counterproductive to the protection of the public.

Following further study and deliberation among the organizations and agencies principally concerned, a final report, published in 1977, limited its recommendations to the allied health professions without including the practice of medicine.[6] Its recommendations included the establishment of a broadly representative national (nongovernmental) certification commission; the development of national standards to determine the credentials for selected health occupations; proposals to be entertained by states to license additional categories of health personnel; steps to be undertaken by states to strengthen the accountability and effectiveness of licensure boards that will allow them to play an active role in assuring quality health services; certification organizations, licensure boards and professional associations to promote the widespread adoption of effective measures to determine the competency of health personnel; and the same agencies to adopt requirements and procedures to assure the continued competence of health personnel.

The staff of the National Board, through its involvement in the examination to evaluate the qualifications for certification for physician's assistants, had obvious interest in the planning for the proposed organization that developed under the aegis of the American Society of Allied Health Professions (ASAHP) and that in December 1977 became established as the National Commission for Health Certifying Agencies. The Board has recommended that testing agencies serve as members on an advisory committee but that they not be members of the organization. This then is another example of the National Board's position in response to a developing problem demonstrating initiatives taken on matters of public policy where the Board has unique insight to offer.

The Future

As a profession, we are facing a future of increasing accountability to the public in terms of medical education, biomedical research, credentials of physicians and associated health care providers, and organization for provision of comprehensive health care. The choice of pathways for the National Board of Medical Examiners is between two major strategies—to be responsive to medical organizations or to exercise initiatives in matters pertaining to public policy. The Board has become more assertive on such issues in recent years and it seems probable that this policy will continue. Some issues which might appropriately and effectively be addressed by the National Board of Medical Examiners in the future are discussed below.

High Scientific Standards vs. Education for Minimum Knowledge—"Intellectualism vs. Relevance"

In the early years of its existence, the goal of the National Board of Medical Examiners was to produce examinations for competency in medicine of such high quality and high stardards that official licensing organizations would accept them in lieu of their own. Members of medical school faculties in the major disciplines were given responsibility for determination of scientific content in the examinations while the staff of the Board working with the subject-matter experts assured that the examinations were reliable measuring instruments. Over the years, medical faculties, recognizing the quality of the National Board examinations, began to use them as measures of educational achievement of their own students. Thus the examinations did not develop as *minimum* competence examinations for licensure, but rather they became tools for rigorous evaluation of student achievement. The difficulty level and the passing grade are above those required as the *minimum* standard for licensure and in fact, should the examinations become the sole route to licensure, it seems likely that the passing standard would have to be lowered at the public's insistence. The National Board has fortunately been in a position to remain independent, insisting on a very high standard of performance for certification of individuals as diplomates. It seems appropriate for the Board with its test committees to continue in its certification role while it simultaneously participates in the development of appropriate minimum competence examinations for licensure with the Federation of State Medical Boards. Thus, as I think about the future thrust of the National Board of Medical Examiners in the public interest, it also seems logical for the Board vigorously to preserve both roles: first as defender of intellectualism and a broad science base in medical education and second as a source of assurance that licensure examinations measure relevant knowledge and skills essential for the safe practice of medicine. The Board could continue to stand as a bulwark against anti-intellectualism while it simultaneously participates in the sound and fair assurance to the public that it is protected against knowledge incompetence in physicians.

Initiatives in Professional Self-discipline

To the extent possible, the Board assures the public and the profession of the integrity of its examinations. It carries the heavy obligation both of searching for evidence of irregular behavior of potential physicians and of reporting such evidence by invalidating scores of knowingly or unknowingly errant students. This obligation carries with it serious risks of litigation against the Board in an area dealing with statistical probabilities—not certainties. The National Board of Medical Examiners must not permit threats of legal action taken to protect an individual's constitutional rights and privileges prevent it from taking action when examination irregularities can be demonstrated. To fail out of fear to take such action would erode our serious obligation to defend the public against possible dishonesty and lack of integrity in its potential physicians.

Relicensure

There is no doubt that the proliferation of essential medical knowledge is such that a physician's fund of knowledge left unattended will surely decay. It is not sensible therefore that a permit to practice medicine awarded at one evaluation point in a physician's career should remain valid for life. The responsibility for licensure lies quite appropriately with state boards of medical licensure. Presently state boards in a growing number of states are insisting on some evidence of physician participation in continuing medical education for reregistration for licensure on a regular basis. Through a variety of methods, physicians should and will insist on the opportunity to show evidence of their "up-to-dateness" to practice in their area of medicine. Evaluation by peer review, chart audit, course participation and examinations are likely mechanisms to be used to document current competence. The National Board is involved in studies to assure that whatever mechanism is used be valid. The Board already is deeply committed to helping organizations in medicine develop self-assessment examinations, physician profiling strategies and recertifying examinations. The Board must stand ready to aid the Federation of State Medical Boards and individual state boards in the development of relicensure examinations appropriate to evaluate individual physicians with widely variable types of practice. It is possible that the Board should take the initiative to both develop and administer for voluntary use an examination appropriate to assess the current competence of practicing physicians. This examination might become acceptable to state boards for relicensure just as the National Board certificate is acceptable for initial licensure and just as the AMA Physician's Recognition Award is used by some states as one option for eligibility for reregistration for licensure. In any case, the National Board of Medical Examiners must continue to evaluate various methods for assessment of the competency of the practicing physician.

Recertification in the Specialties

The 22 primary specialty boards all have agreed in principle with the logic of some system of certification renewal.[7] Some have already decided that recertification should be mandatory and that certification in the future will be awarded to cover a specified time. The National Board is working with specialty boards as they try to define criteria for documenting continuing competence through recertification. Studies of methods of profiling of specialists according to type of practice is but one of the areas of relevant investigation being pursued. Validation of chart audit methods, behavioral checklists, simulation techniques and computer-based examinations may bear on methods which specialty boards will find useful in the years ahead. In the era of recertification the National Board's role is and should continue to be serving the specialty boards and helping them to develop the most valid evaluation programs possible for recertification.

Initiatives to Effect Public (Government) Health Policy

Although there is no way accurately to predict the future initiatives which will be taken by the federal government in relation to medical practice, the National Board of Medical Examiners must assert itself to influence favorably those measures which are sensible, logical and achievable in the public interest. At the same time, the Board is in a unique position to recognize that some federal proposals which seem reasonable to legislators will in fact be counterproductive and in the end detrimental to the public interest. The National Board must remain well informed on federal initiatives and must stand ready to react to them, to urge modification or dissolution of propositions that may do disservice to the public and to the profession.

Commitment to Education in Evaluation of Professional Competence

Although the preamble of the National Board bylaws (as revised in 1967) indicates the appropriateness of the Board's offering educational opportunities to individuals wishing to study methods, techniques and value of testing methods related to knowledge and competence in medicine, there has not as yet been any formal National Board fellowship program for such individuals. Many professionals from around the world have visited the Board for various intervals on an ad hoc basis. In 1976, the Board in adopting the recommendations of its Policy Advisory Committee[8] approved the principle of developing formal educational programs to aid those interested in developing evaluation expertise. In the years ahead the National Board should offer its intrinsic expertise to increase the number of professionals qualified to participate in upgrading evaluation of medical competence around the world. It is self-evident that the public interest would be well served by such an effort.

Initiatives in International Exchange of Materials, Methods and Credentials

The Annual Conference of the National Board in March 1976, entitled An International View of Qualification for the Practice of Medicine, was devoted to a discussion by international figures in the evaluation field of the ways in which interrelationships and exchange of information might profit the international public.[9] As the world exchange increases with modern communications and transportation, it is inevitable that multinational cooperation among credentialing and testing agencies must occur. The National Board should not only welcome but initiate exchanges with counterpart organizations around the world with the purpose of upgrading and helping to standardize the qualifications for medical practice.

Summary

These and other issues constitute areas where the National Board in the years ahead may have the opportunity to wield a strong positive influence. The National Board of Medical Examiners is a fundamental part of organized medicine, and in a generic sense it should take the responsibility to prepare itself to respond to public pressures—both national and international—for the development of standards in evaluation and common evaluation procedures.

References

1. Stevens, R. A.: The National Board and the Public Interest. The National Board Examiner, Vol. 19, No 8, May 1972.
2. Evaluation in the Continuum of Medical Education. Report of the Committee on Goals and Priorities of the National Board of Medical Examiners (Mayer, W. D., Chairman). National Board of Medical Examiners, Philadelphia, 1973.
3. The Graduate Education of Physicians. Report of the Citizens Commission on Graduate Medical Education (John S. Millis, Chairman). American Medical Association, Chicago, 1966.
4. Higher Education and the Nation's Health. Report of the Carnegie Commission on Higher Education. McGraw-Hill, New York, 1970.
5. A Proposal for Credentialing Health Manpower. Report of the Subcommittee on Health Manpower Credentialing of the Public Health Service Health Manpower Coordinating Committee (Cohen, H. S., Chairman). Department of Health, Education and Welfare, Washington, June 1976.
6. Credentialling Health Manpower. Publication No. (OS) 77-50057. Department of Health, Education and Welfare, Washington, July 1977.
7. Leymaster, G. R. (Ed): American Board of Medical Specialties Annual Report 1976–77. American Board of Medical Specialties, Chicago, 1977.
8. Levit, E. J. (Ed.): Report of the Policy Advisory Committee of the National Board of Medical Examiners (Holden, W. D., Chairman). National Board of Medical Examiners, Philadelphia, March 1976.
9. Annual Conference of the National Board of Medical Examiners: An International View of the Qualifications for Medical Practice. Philadelphia, March 1976.

APPENDIX A

■

Senior Staff of the National Board of Medical Examiners (January 1978)

Edithe J. Levit, M.D., President and Director
David E. Smith, M.D., Vice-President and Secretary
Fredric D. Burg, M.D., Vice-President
Alice J. Wooden, Assistant to the President
Department of Undergraduate Medical Evaluation
David E. Smith, M.D., Director
William B. Kennedy, M.D., Co-Director
Bryce Templeton, M.D., Project Director, CQE
Ethel Weinberg, M.D., Associate Director
Robert H. Schussel, Ph.D., Assistant Director
Judith L. McGuire, Editorial Supervisor and Coordinator TIL Project
Department of Graduate and Continuing Medical Evaluation
Fredric D. Burg, M.D., Director
Paul Lee Brading, Ph.D., Associate Director
Norris R. Culf, M.D.
Robert O. Guerin, Ph.D., Assistant Director
Victor C. Vaughan, Senior Evaluation Fellow
Department of Research and Development
Barbara J. Andrew, Ph.D., Director
Vivian F. Erviti, Ph.D., Associate Director
Thomas Samph, Ph.D., Associate Director
Edgar L. Richards, Ph.D., Assistant Director
Department of Psychometrics
Charles F. Schumacher, Ph.D., Director
Paul R. Kelley, Jr., Ph.D., Co-Director
Martin E. Grosse, Ph.D., Associate Director
Francis P. Hughes, Ph.D., Associate Director
Anita I. Bell, Ph. D., Assistant Director
Department of Finance and Administration
William L. Slobodnik, Director
Robert J. Campbell, Data Processing Systems and Operations Director

Richard C. Barth, Data Processing Manager
Thomas L. Williams, Systems and Programming Manager
David C. Kreines, Systems Analyst
Nicholas L. Luongo, Data Processing Standards and Software Support
    Manager
Thomas J. Conway, Systems Programmer
Eugene R. Keller, Administrative Services Manager
John T. Wosnitzer, Financial Manager
Jeannette B. Massias, Controller
Thomas R. Belvedere, Production Manager
Mildred E. Wesner, Test Administration Manager
Ann K. Heverling, Registrar and Secretary for Certification

APPENDIX B

■

Examples of Test Questions Used in Examinations of the National Board of Medical Examiners

The following test questions are examples of those used in National Board examinations, and have been drawn from the Board's collection of calibrated test questions. Each of the types (forms) of multiple-choice questions in current use is represented by one or more examples.

One hundred questions have been selected from the seven traditional basic medical sciences (Part I): anatomy, behavioral sciences, biochemistry, microbiology, pathology, pharmacology and physiology; 100 from the six clinical subjects (Part II): internal medicine, obstetrics and gynecology, pediatrics, preventive medicine and public health, psychiatry and surgery. Additional questions used and tested in the Part III examination illustrate the use of pictorial material in each of the three parts of the National Board's examinations. A set of patient management problems demonstrates the special feature of the Part III examination familiarly known as PMP (see Chapter 4).

The set of 100 questions in the basic medical sciences and that in the clinical subjects are not to be mistaken for full Part I and Part II examinations. They are presented here to demonstrate the methodology of National Board examinations, not as an example of well-rounded or balanced content. A test of 100 multiple-choice questions would normally take 1½ hours. Part I and Part II consist of about 900 to 1000 test questions respectively, scheduled for totals of 12 and 13 hours.

Based upon the item analysis derived from the use of these questions for National Board candidates, the difficulty of the abbreviated sample "test," expressed as the average number of times each item was answered correctly by the candidates and spoken of as the mean P value (see page 51), and the effectiveness of the test in discriminating the high-scoring from the low-scoring group of candidates, referred to as the r index (see page 52), have been calculated for each set of 100 items.

	Mean P valve	Mean r index
100 Basic Science Questions	.68	.37
100 Clinical Questions	.67	.35

The difficulty level of each of these two sample tests is close to that of National Board examinations, where the mean P value is usually in the range of .60 to .65. The mean r index for these two sets of questions, .37 and .35, respectively, is somewhat higher than that expected for a complete Part I or Part II examination because, in these sample tests, only questions that have performed well when used have been selected, whereas the full Part I and Part II examinations are newly constructed each year and are largely made up of test questions not yet put to the test of usage.

The few examples of pictorial material are taken from a section of the Part III examination that would usually contain approximately 130 test questions scheduled for a 2½-hour examination. These examples, however, are sufficient to give some impression of the versatility of this testing method in contrast to the "slide quiz" familiar to several of the American specialty boards, where the candidate has a few predetermined seconds or minutes to view one picture at a time as projected on a screen; he cannot compare one picture with another as when, for example, a series of blood smears is printed in the test booklet as the basis for a differential diagnosis or when, as demonstrated in these samples, a series of electrocardiograms is the basis for several questions.

The set of patient management problems (PMP) related to a single patient demonstrates the testing method forming the main part of the single day scheduled for Part III. In the actual examination, the candidate would encounter as many as 20 such sets, each containing 2 to 5 problems, for a testing session of 3½ or 4 hours. Since this testing technique is less familiar than that of multiple-choice questions, carefully worded and detailed instructions are printed on the cover of the test book and time is allowed for the examinees to study these instructions carefully.

When the PMP test is printed for use in an examination, a block of chemically sensitized material covers each response to hide the information given for the result of a selected choice of action. The examinee must then develop this block with a special "pen" that is provided in order to reveal the result of the decision. (For purposes of this demonstration, the responses that would underlie the blocks are provided at the end of the section.) To obtain a fair impression of the task involved in taking this test, the reader should endeavor to look only at the response for the single choice of action selected before making the next choice and looking at the next response.

In the instructions preceding the test, candidates are informed that, in scoring these problems, they are given credit for correct choices (selecting and developing indicated options and leaving undeveloped those that are not appropriate) and are thus penalized for errors of commission (selecting incorrect courses of action) and omission (failing to select correct courses of action).

When the PMP included here was used in a Part III examination, the average National Board candidate made 30 correct choices and 13 incorrect choices.

**Part I—Examples of Questions Drawn From Basic-Science Subjects:
Questions 1–100**

DIRECTIONS: Each of the questions or incomplete statements below is followed by five suggested answers or completions. Select the <u>one</u> that is BEST in each case.

1. Which of the following veins is a part of a portal system?

    (A) Right ovarian
    (B) Left ovarian
    (C) Middle rectal
    (D) Superior rectal
    (E) Uterine

2. Sinusoids interposed between two sets of veins are found in the

    (A) small intestine
    (B) spleen
    (C) anterior pituitary gland
    (D) placenta
    (E) parathyroid glands

3. The edema of acute inflammation involves the exudation of protein-rich fluid

    (A) primarily through venules and capillaries
    (B) primarily through arterioles
    (C) only through capillaries
    (D) through lymphatic vessels
    (E) through all microvessels more or less equally

4. A factor responsible for edema in the nephrotic syndrome is

    (A) increased filtration pressure of the blood plasma
    (B) decreased osmotic pressure of the blood plasma
    (C) decreased capillary permeability
    (D) retention of potassium
    (E) increased blood lipids

5. Carbon dioxide is transported in the blood primarily as

    (A) dissolved CO_2
    (B) carbonic acid
    (C) carbaminohemoglobin
    (D) plasma bicarbonate
    (E) intracellular bicarbonate in red blood cells

6. The release of carbon dioxide from blood in pulmonary capillaries is retarded by

    (A) the simultaneous absorption of oxygen
    (B) any increase in the alveolar carbon-dioxide tension
    (C) carbonic anhydrase
    (D) the chloride shift
    (E) the buffer effect of hemoglobin

7. A molar solution of an electrolyte has a higher osmotic pressure than a molar solution of a nonelectrolyte because the

    (A) electrolyte ions carry electric charges
    (B) electrolyte ions are usually hydrated
    (C) electrolyte alters the dielectric constant of water
    (D) electrolyte dissociates in solution
    (E) nonelectrolyte is not polar

8. Sustained motivated forgetting is

    (A) reaction formation
    (B) projection
    (C) repression
    (D) intellectualization
    (E) regression

9. The fourth cranial or trochlear nerve innervates

    (A) the lacrimal gland
    (B) a muscle that turns the eyeball superiorly and laterally
    (C) the medial part of the lower eyelid
    (D) a muscle that turns the eyeball inferiorly and laterally
    (E) the lacrimal caruncle

10. A patient's left upper eyelid droops, his left eyeball is apparently recessed, and his left pupil is constricted. The left side of his face is flushed but dry. Which of the following is the most likely diagnosis?

    (A) A tumor in the interpeduncular fossa pressing forward on the posterior hypothalamic nuclei and backward on the left oculomotor nerve
    (B) A tumor in the pretectal region
    (C) A tumor pressing on the cervical sympathetic trunk
    (D) An infarct of the branch of the middle cerebral artery supplying the middle region of the precentral gyrus of the frontal lobe
    (E) None of the above

11. In basal fractures of the skull, if cerebrospinal fluid escapes from the nose, there is probably a fracture of the

    (A) nasal bone
    (B) temporal bone
    (C) ethmoid bone
    (D) parietal bone
    (E) frontal bone

12. If a patient has received no preanesthetic medication and breathes a gas mixture of 80 per cent nitrous oxide and 20 per cent oxygen, which of the following is most likely to occur?

    (A) Severe damage to the brain, consequent to anoxia
    (B) Analgesia
    (C) Deep surgical anesthesia
    (D) Respiratory arrest
    (E) No obvious effect

13. Spinal transection at about T6 may be followed by hypotension resulting primarily from

    (A) impairment of sympathetic vasoconstriction
    (B) impairment of myocardial contraction
    (C) lack of proprioceptive input from the lower limbs
    (D) a decrease in the volume of circulating whole blood
    (E) none of the above

14. Loss of scattered anterior horn cells by amyotrophic lateral sclerosis results in which of the following changes in a skeletal muscle such as the deltoid?

        (A) Atrophy of single muscle fibers
        (B) Atrophy of muscle fibers of individual motor units
        (C) Diffuse atrophy of muscle fibers
        (D) Swelling and hyalinization of muscle fibers
        (E) Regenerative buds and increased sarcolemmal nuclei

15. In progressive muscular dystrophy, the essential pathological changes occur

        (A) in anterior horn cells of the spinal cord
        (B) in motor fibers of peripheral nerves
        (C) in motor end-plates (myoneural junctions)
        (D) within muscle fibers
        (E) in the ground substance of muscular interstitium

16. In both sexes

        (A) the bladder in adults is confined to the true pelvis (pelvis minor)
        (B) the major source of blood to the rectum is from the middle rectal (hemorrhoidal) arteries
        (C) the small intestine may be in contact with the bladder (through peritoneum)
        (D) the median sacral artery cannot be ligated without serious effects
        (E) efferent (motor) fibers from the sacral levels of the spinal cord pass directly to the muscle of the bladder

17. The phenomenon of "imprinting" is primarily dependent upon the

        (A) type of environment
        (B) age of the subject
        (C) stimulus presented
        (D) number of siblings present
        (E) age of the parents

18. When a person engages in behavior that is inconsistent with a previously held attitude, a motivational state will be aroused that can pressure the individual to change his attitude so as to make it more consistent with his behavior. The state is termed

>   (A) central efferent process
>   (B) stimulus manipulation
>   (C) orienting reflex
>   (D) temporal integration
>   (E) cognitive dissonance

19. Death in diphtheria is usually caused by

>   (A) laryngeal paralysis
>   (B) hyperthermia
>   (C) convulsions with brain damage
>   (D) respiratory failure
>   (E) myocardial failure

20. Which of the following processes is most likely to predispose to the development of a tubal pregnancy?

>   (A) Tuberculous endometritis
>   (B) Vaginitis related to trichomoniasis
>   (C) Lymphopathia venereum
>   (D) Syphilis
>   (E) Gonococcal salpingitis

21. The bacterium that most frequently causes meningitis with a predominance of lymphocytes in spinal fluid is

>   (A) *Neisseria meningitidis*
>   (B) *Haemophilus influenzae*
>   (C) *Staphylococcus aureus*
>   (D) *Mycobacterium tuberculosis*
>   (E) *Streptococcus pneumoniae*

22. The most practicable available method for controlling the spread of St. Louis encephalitis virus is

>   (A) eradication of wild waterfowl
>   (B) eradication of houseflies
>   (C) vaccination of poultry flocks
>   (D) intensive mosquito control
>   (E) burning over marshlands

23. The principal reason for administering live poliovirus vaccine on a 3-dose schedule is to

        (A) reduce the chance of interference among poliovirus types
        (B) provide a booster or anamnestic response
        (C) lessen neurotoxicity
        (D) permit continued clinical surveillance of the recipient
        (E) increase the opportunity for viral interference with wild-type enteroviruses

24. The effectiveness of interferon as an antiviral agent depends upon its ability to

        (A) combine with and neutralize extracellular virions
        (B) prevent the penetration of viruses into a cell
        (C) destroy the protein coat surrounding a virus
        (D) act intracellularly to prevent the production of new mature virions
        (E) stimulate the host defenses, leading to earlier and increased antibody production

25. The ineffectiveness of penicillins against fungi, protozoa, and viruses can be attributed to the

        (A) lack of sterols in membranes or envelopes
        (B) presence of sterols in membranes or envelopes
        (C) impermeability of cell membranes to penicillin
        (D) absence of mucopeptide-containing cell walls
        (E) production of penicillinase by these organisms

26. The basis for the toxic action of the polyene antibiotics (nystatin and amphotericin B) on microorganisms is dependent upon their binding to

        (A) sterols
        (B) lipoproteins
        (C) chitin
        (D) nucleic acids
        (E) polysaccharides

27. Complement is required in order to demonstrate

    (A) immune bacteriolysis
    (B) heterophil sheep-cell agglutination
    (C) the agar gel diffusion reaction
    (D) typhoid O agglutinins
    (E) diphtheria toxin-antitoxin flocculation

28. The mechanism by which antihistaminic compounds relieve allergic conditions involves

    (A) acceleration of the excretion of histamine
    (B) neutralization of the effects of histamine by producing the opposite reactions
    (C) chemical combination with histamine and inactivation of it
    (D) competition with histamine in attachment to cell receptors
    (E) activation of histamine oxidase

29. Concerning the effects of various means of communication, it has generally been found that

    (A) there is no consistent difference between written and oral messages
    (B) written messages tend to be both better comprehended and more persuasive than do the same messages presented orally
    (C) oral messages tend to be both better comprehended and more persuasive than do the same messages presented in writing
    (D) although oral messages tend to be better comprehended than written messages, the latter tend to have a more persuasive impact
    (E) although written messages tend to be better comprehended than oral messages, the latter tend to have a more persuasive impact

30. Administration of luteinizing hormone to a male causes

    (A) increased spermatogenesis
    (B) stimulation of androgen secretion by cells of the seminiferous tubules
    (C) secretion of androgen by interstitial cells of the testes
    (D) contraction of the epididymis
    (E) increased motility of Leydig's cells

DIRECTIONS: This section of the test consists of situations, each followed by a series of questions. Study each situation, and select the one best answer to each question following it.

Questions 31–34

A 68-year-old physician, apparently well except for mild diabetes mellitus and essential hypertension (blood pressure 160/95 mm Hg), both of about 10 years' duration, felt severe crushing precordial pain while shoveling snow. He collapsed and was taken to a hospital, where he was found to be in shock and cyanotic with hypotension and a rapid, feeble pulse. Given oxygen and supportive therapy, he improved somewhat, his blood pressure returning to its former level. Six days after admission, while using the bed pan, the patient died suddenly. At autopsy, extensive myocardial infarction was found.

31. Examination of the kidneys would be most likely to disclose

   (A) acute pyelonephritis
   (B) acute glomerulonephritis
   (C) benign nephrosclerosis
   (D) malignant nephrosclerosis
   (E) chronic glomerulonephritis

32. The most likely cause of the myocardial infarction was

   (A) syphilitic aortitis with occlusion of a coronary orifice
   (B) embolus to a coronary artery
   (C) dissecting aneurysm with occlusion of a coronary orifice
   (D) occlusion of a coronary orifice due to atheroma
   (E) coronary thrombus on the basis of an atheroma

33. Histologically, the prominent feature of the infarct might have been any of the following EXCEPT

   (A) necrotic muscle
   (B) infiltration by polymorphonuclear leukocytes
   (C) replacement of muscle by fibrous tissue
   (D) fibrinous exudate on the pericardium
   (E) unorganized endocardial thrombus

34. One might expect to find each of the following EXCEPT

   (A) fibrinous pericarditis
   (B) verrucous endocarditis
   (C) endocardial thrombus
   (D) rupture of the myocardium
   (E) cardiac dilatation

Questions 35–39

An overdose of a new drug produced progressive effects referable to the central nervous system including vertigo, ataxia, somnolence, hypnosis and respiratory depression. These began within 15 minutes after oral administration of the drug. No metabolic breakdown products were found in the urine; however, a high concentration of the agent was found in the bile.

The following information was obtained from the manufacturer: The drug is an organic acid with a pK_a of 6.4 and high lipid solubility; the drug is excreted by humans in such a way that one half of the administered drug is eliminated in the urine within three days.

35. The symptoms and physicochemical data indicate that the drug probably

    (A) passes readily through cell membranes, including the blood-brain barrier

    (B) passes readily through cell membranes but does not pass the blood-brain barrier

    (C) penetrates readily from the circulation into the brain but not into other organs

    (D) can diffuse only into the glomerular filtrate

    (E) cannot escape from the circulation

36. The information that the drug is highly concentrated in bile suggests

    (A) that the drug is probably efficiently excreted in the feces

    (B) that the drug is probably structurally similar to a bile acid

    (C) that the drug forms complexes with bile acids

    (D) that the drug is effectively absorbed from the large intestine

    (E) none of the above conclusions

37. The fact that it takes three days for half of the drug to appear in the urine is best explained on the basis that the drug

    (A) is bound to plasma protein

    (B) undergoes little or no metabolism and is passively reabsorbed from the renal tubules

    (C) is deposited in bone

    (D) is actively secreted by the renal tubules

    (E) does none of the above

38. The ratio of the unionized to the ionized form of the drug in plasma at pH 7.4 is

> (A) 1:10
> (B) 1:1
> (C) 10:1
> (D) 100:1
> (E) 1000:1

39. Acidification of the urine by administration of ammonium sulfate would

> (A) increase the relative concentration of the ionized form of the drug in tubular fluid, which is likely to increase urinary excretion
> (B) increase the relative concentration of the ionized form of the drug, which is likely to decrease urinary excretion
> (C) decrease the relative concentration of the ionized form of the drug, which is likely to increase urinary excretion
> (D) decrease the relative concentration of the ionized form of the drug, which is likely to decrease urinary excretion
> (E) increase secretion of the drug by the renal tubules

Questions 40–42

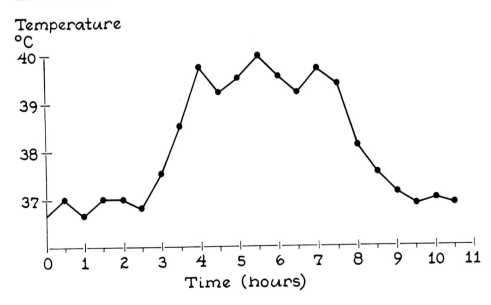

The figure above shows the time course of a typical febrile episode as recorded from a rectal thermometer.

40. During the onset of the febrile period,

    (A) the elevation in body temperature is promptly sensed by hypothalamic thermal receptors that activate cooling mechanisms
    (B) cutaneous warm receptors are relatively active
    (C) sweating and vasodilation appear promptly
    (D) the patient responds physiologically through mechanisms ordinarily activated by a cold environment
    (E) a breakdown in thermogenesis takes place

41. During the period of sustained fever,

    (A) regulatory adjustments are maintained but are less precise
    (B) heat production steadily exceeds heat loss
    (C) total heat loss steadily exceeds heat production
    (D) radiative and convective heat losses are markedly reduced
    (E) the hypothalamic "thermostat" is reset at an abnormally low value

42. In producing fever of this type, endogenous pyrogens in the blood

    (A) act upon skeletal muscle to increase metabolic activity
    (B) directly inhibit secretory activity of the sweat glands
    (C) directly induce both shivering and vasodilation
    (D) act to reset the hypothalamic "thermostat" to regulate at a higher temperature
    (E) directly attack and destroy infectious disease organisms

---

DIRECTIONS: Each group of questions below consists of five lettered headings or a diagram or table with five lettered components, followed by a list of numbered words, phrases or statements. For <u>each</u> numbered word, phrase or statement, select the <u>one</u> lettered heading or lettered component that is most closely associated with it. Each lettered heading or lettered component may be selected once, more than once, or not at all.

Questions 43–45

For each region, indicate the epithelium that would usually be expected.

    (A) Stratified squamous
    (B) Transitional
    (C) Simple columnar
    (D) Simple cuboidal
    (E) Pseudostratified ciliated columnar

43. The primary bronchus

44. The ileocolic junction

45. The proximal part of the female urethra

Questions 46–48

    (A) Bacterial flagellum
    (B) Mitochondrion
    (C) Cell membrane
    (D) Wall of a gram-positive bacterium
    (E) Wall of a gram-negative bacterium

46. The location of cytochrome enzymes in bacteria

47. The location of teichoic acids

48. An entity composed exclusively of protein

Questions 49–51

    (A) Amphotericin B
    (B) Nystatin
    (C) Neomycin
    (D) Griseofulvin
    (E) Bacitracin

49. An antifungal agent effective in the treatment of systemic mycoses

50. An antifungal agent effective in the treatment of ringworm of the skin and nails

51. An agent used primarily in the treatment of *Candida* infections of the skin, mucous membrane and intestinal tract

Questions 52–54

    (A) Nitrogen mustard
    (B) ^{32}P
    (C) Methotrexate (Amethopterin)
    (D) 6-Mercaptopurine
    (E) Colchicine

52. A hypoxanthine analog

53. An agent which interrupts mitotic activity at the metaphase

54. An alkylating agent

Questions 55–58

Patient	Distressful Signs or Symptoms	Respiratory Minute Vol. (l/minute)	Urinary pH	Urinary 24-Hour Vol. (ml)	Na^+	Plasma (mEq/l) K^+	Cl^-	HCO_3^-
Normal	None	8	6.8	2000	140	5	100	27
(A)	Shortness of breath	5	6.0	2100	141	5.1	94	34
(B)	Weakness	7.8	7.3	1800	129	7	92	26
(C)	Hyperpnea	10	5.8	4000	124	5.1	90	11
(D)	Dizziness and muscle twitching	16	7.6	2200	134	4.9	105	22
(E)	Thirst	8	7.2	15,000	165	5.5	125	27

The table above presents information concerning the respiratory, renal and acid-base states of several different patients in relation to values approximating those found in normal men. For each question, select the letter designating the patient most likely to be represented by the situation described.

55. The patient has a plasma pH significantly greater than normal

56. The patient is experiencing interference with the free movement of air in respiratory passageways

57. The patient has been experiencing excessive metabolic production of acids, such as acetoacetic acid, possibly due to unregulated diabetes mellitus

58. The patient has an inadequately functioning posterior pituitary gland

Questions 59–62

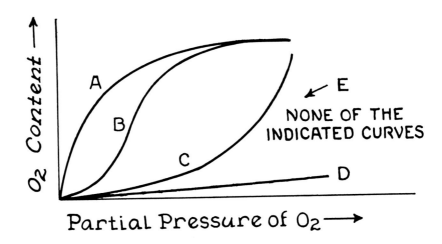

Each of the lettered curves shown above may depict a relationship of the total content of oxygen in solution to the partial pressure of oxygen.

59. Shape of the curve that represents the relationship of oxygen contained in physical solution in plasma to the partial pressure of oxygen

60. Shape of the curve that would be observed for the reversible binding of oxygen to normal human myoglobin

61. Shape of the curve that would be observed for the reversible binding of oxygen to normal human hemoglobin

62. Shape of the curve that would be observed for the binding of oxygen to an abnormal human hemoglobin that lacks heme-heme interaction

Questions 63–67

DIRECTION OF ARROW indicates change from average normal values; 0 indicates absence of change from normal.

	ARTERIAL BLOOD		MIXED VENOUS BLOOD	
	O_2 content ml/100 ml	P_{O_2} mm Hg	O_2 content ml/100 ml	P_{O_2} mm Hg
(A)	↓	↓	↓	↓
(B)	0	0	↑	↑
(C)	↓	↑	↓	↓
(D)	↑	↑	↓	↓
(E)	↓	0	↓	↓

63. Iron-deficiency anemia

64. A femoral arteriovenous fistula

65. Acute respiratory failure in poliomyelitis

66. Nonfatal carbon-monoxide poisoning

67. Severe barbiturate poisoning

Questions 68–71

A study of intermediary metabolism has revealed that most vitamins function as the precursors of coenzymes or prosthetic groups. For each numbered item, select the vitamin involved in its formation.

(A) Thiamine
(B) Nicotinamide
(C) Vitamin C
(D) Vitamin B_6
(E) Pantothenic acid

68. Diphosphopyridine nucleotide

69. Pyridoxal phosphate

70. Cocarboxylase

71. Coenzyme A

DIRECTIONS: Each set of lettered headings below is followed by a list of numbered words or phrases. For each numbered word or phrase select

A if the item is associated with (A) only,
B if the item is associated with (B) only,
C if the item is associated with both (A) and (B),
D if the item is associated with neither (A) nor (B).

Questions 72–75

(A) Cellular proliferation continually renews the cellular population in adults
(B) Cellular proliferation occurs or increases sporadically to compensate for injury or to meet increased functional demands
(C) Both
(D) Neither

72. Neurons

73. Intestinal absorptive cells

74. Hepatic parenchymal cells

75. Epidermis

Questions 76–78

    (A) Chronic myelocytic leukemia
    (B) Acute myeloblastic leukemia
    (C) Both
    (D) Neither

76. Chromosomal errors in leukemic cells

77. Ph¹ (Philadelphia) chromosome (G group deletion)

78. Down's syndrome (mongolism)

DIRECTIONS: For each of the questions or incomplete statements below, ONE or MORE of the answers or completions given is correct. Select

    A if only 1, 2, and 3 are correct,
    B if only 1 and 3 are correct,
    C if only 2 and 4 are correct,
    D if only 4 is correct,
    E if all are correct.

Directions Summarized				
A	B	C	D	E
1,2,3 only	1,3 only	2,4 only	4 only	All are correct

79. The molecular weight of a protein may be estimated by

    (1) infrared analysis
    (2) ultracentrifugation
    (3) electrophoresis
    (4) gel filtration

80. Forces or bonds that may be important in determining the three-dimensional structure of proteins include

    (1) covalent bonds
    (2) electrostatic attraction and repulsion forces
    (3) hydrogen bonds
    (4) hydrophobic bonds

81. The immunogenicity of macromolecules generally

    (1) is greatest for proteins
    (2) involves the recognition of the macromolecule as foreign to the host
    (3) depends on the route of administration
    (4) is enhanced by prior enzymatic fragmentation

82. Subcutaneous injections of one's own tissues from which of the following would induce the production of autoantibodies?

    (1) Brain
    (2) Thyroid
    (3) Spermatozoa
    (4) Uterine muscle

83. A reaction of the delayed type occurs in the

    (1) tuberculin skin test
    (2) Schick test
    (3) mumps skin test
    (4) ragweed pollen skin test

84. The classical Arthus' reaction is associated with

    (1) the presence of precipitating antibodies
    (2) migration of polymorphonuclear leukocytes to the reaction site
    (3) fixation of complement to the antigen-antibody aggregate
    (4) histamine release

85. Genetic resistance of bacteria to antibiotics can be acquired by

    (1) the uptake of DNA extracted from resistant cells of the same species
    (2) phage-mediated transduction from resistant donors
    (3) the conjugational transfer of an episome
    (4) mutation specifically induced by the antibiotic

Directions Summarized				
A	B	C	D	E
1,2,3	1,3	2,4	4	All are
only	only	only	only	correct

86. Cholera is characterized by

    (1) liquid stools low in protein and high in potassium and bicar-
        bonate
    (2) hemoconcentration, acidosis, and hypokalemia
    (3) paralysis of the sodium-potassium pump of the intestinal
        mucosa
    (4) blood cultures positive for *Vibrio cholerae*

87. Capsules of *Streptococcus pneumoniae*

    (1) consist of lipopolysaccharide, protein, and carbohydrate
    (2) stimulate the formation of protective antibodies
    (3) are most likely to be found on pneumococci grown in the
        presence of type-specific antipneumococcal antibody
    (4) are required for virulence

88. Reactions in which there is a net loss of an energy-rich phosphate bond
    include

    (1) 1,3-diphosphoglyceric acid + $H_2O \rightarrow$ 3-phosphoglyceric acid
        + inorganic phosphate
    (2) ATP + creatine $\rightarrow$ creatine-phosphate + ADP
    (3) ATP + glucose $\rightarrow$ glucose-6-phosphate + ADP
    (4) 2-ADP $\rightarrow$ ATP + AMP

89. In Type I glycogen storage disease (glucose-6-phosphate deficiency),
    there is an abnormally large accumulation of glycogen in the

    (1) liver
    (2) cardiac muscle
    (3) kidneys
    (4) skeletal muscle

Directions Summarized				
A	B	C	D	E
1,2,3 only	1,3 only	2,4 only	4 only	All are correct

90. Enzymes

    (1) increase the rate of a reaction
    (2) lower the activation energy of a reaction
    (3) act specifically on one substrate or a group of related substrates
    (4) alter the equilibrium constant of a reaction

91. The pK_a of lactic acid is 3.85. A buffer could be prepared at this pH by the addition of

    (1) 50 ml of 0.1 N sodium hydroxide to 100 ml of 0.1 N lactic acid
    (2) 100 ml 0.1 N sodium lactate to 50 ml of 0.2 N lactic acid
    (3) 50 ml of 0.2 N sodium lactate to 50 ml of 0.1 N hydrochloric acid
    (4) 50 ml of 0.2 N sodium hydroxide to 50 ml of 0.1 N lactic acid

92. The major mechanisms for the termination of norepinephrine action in the body include

    (1) methylation to 3-methoxy-norepinephrine (normetanephrine) by the enzyme catechol-O-methyl transferase (COMT)
    (2) deamination to 3,4-dihydroxymandelic acid by the enzyme monoamine oxidase (MAO)
    (3) uptake by nerve endings
    (4) N-methylation to epinephrine

93. Extracts of the hypothalamus act on the pituitary gland to

    (1) increase the output of ACTH
    (2) increase the uptake of ^{131}I by the thyroid gland by increasing the output of thyroid-stimulating hormone
    (3) stimulate ovulation from mature follicles by increasing the output of luteinizing hormone
    (4) decrease the output of prolactin

Directions Summarized				
A	B	C	D	E
1,2,3 only	1,3 only	2,4 only	4 only	All are correct

94. In a population in which there are many poor people and few very rich people, the

    (1) standard deviation of income will be small
    (2) distribution of incomes will be likely to conform to a normal distribution
    (3) modal income will be higher than the mean income
    (4) mean income will be higher than the median income

95. Accumulation of fat in hepatic parenchymal cells can be induced by

    (1) a dietary deficiency of lipotropic factors
    (2) protein deficiency
    (3) ingestion of halogenated hydrocarbons
    (4) chronic ingestion of alcohol

96. Mesoderm in the early embryo is the germ layer source of

    (1) macrophages
    (2) lung epithelium
    (3) pericardium
    (4) hair follicles

97. In the mammalian kidney, urea

    (1) is freely filtrable at the glomerulus
    (2) is actively transported into the proximal tubule
    (3) has a clearance less than that of insulin
    (4) is excreted at a rate independent of the rate of urine flow

98. An ethnic group is a collection of persons considered both by themselves and by others to have one or more of certain characteristics in common. These characteristics include

    (1) religion
    (2) racial origin
    (3) national origin
    (4) language and cultural traditions

A	B	C	D	E
1,2,3 only	1,3 only	2,4 only	4 only	All are correct

Directions Summarized

99. Which of the following vessels usually anastomose with one another and together form a chief supply to the parts named?

   (1) The right gastric and the left gastric arteries supplying the lesser curvature of the stomach
   (2) The superior pancreaticoduodenal and the inferior pancreaticoduodenal arteries supplying the tail of the pancreas
   (3) The right colic artery and the ileocolic artery supplying the appendix
   (4) The left colic artery and the middle colic artery supplying the right (hepatic) flexure of the large intestine

100. Toxic doses of digitoxin may produce

   (1) anorexia
   (2) disturbances of color vision
   (3) ventricular extrasystoles
   (4) vomiting

Part II—Examples of Questions Drawn From Clinical Subjects: Questions 1–100

DIRECTIONS: Each of the questions or incomplete statements below is followed by five suggested answers or completions. Select the one that is BEST in each case.

1. The life expectancy for white females born in 1960 was 73 years. This means that

   (A) the average age at death among white females in 1960 was 73 years
   (B) the life span of white females in 1960 was 73 years
   (C) under mortality conditions in 1960, every white female may expect to live at least 73 years
   (D) the average life expectancy of white females at all ages in 1960 was 73 years
   (E) on the average, white females would live 73 years if the age-specific death rates for white females in 1960 continue unchanged throughout their lives

2. Life expectancy has increased markedly in the United States during the past 50 years chiefly because of

   (A) a continued reduction in the death rates of infants and children
   (B) the continuous decline in tuberculosis
   (C) the fact that older adults reach retirement age in better health
   (D) a fairly uniform reduction of death rates in all age groups
   (E) control of industrial health hazards

3. In acute intestinal obstruction due to incarcerated hernia, the spasms of pain result from

   (A) constriction of the bowel at the site of obstruction
   (B) necrosis of the bowel at the site of obstruction
   (C) inflammatory exudate soiling the peritoneal surfaces
   (D) contraction of the distended bowel above the site of obstruction
   (E) compression of the nerves of the bowel

4. A patient with a history of fever and mild diarrhea of two months' duration is found to have a palpable mass in the right lower quadrant of the abdomen. The most likely diagnosis is

     (A) regional enteritis
     (B) ulcerative colitis
     (C) amebic colitis
     (D) diverticulitis
     (E) lymphoma

5. Uterine retroversion is

     (A) often a cause of pelvic pain
     (B) relatively infrequent
     (C) usually associated with a lumbar backache
     (D) usually asymptomatic
     (E) a cause of endometriosis

6. The decline in the reported deaths from cancer of the stomach is most likely to be the result of

     (A) improved methods of treatment
     (B) changes in death certificate classification
     (C) earlier diagnosis
     (D) lower incidence
     (E) none of the above

7. A 22-year-old multipara, who has had a successful removal of a small intraepithelial carcinoma of the cervix by wide conization, would like to have more children. Management should consist of

     (A) regular pelvic examinations and Papanicolaou smears
     (B) small amounts of radium therapy to the cervix with the ovaries shielded
     (C) annual curettage
     (D) cervical amputation
     (E) administration of progesterone

8. Which of the following, if persistent, is usually incompatible with spontaneous delivery at term?

     (A) Mentum posterior
     (B) Mentum anterior
     (C) Sacrum posterior
     (D) Occiput posterior
     (E) Caput succedaneum

9. Of the following, primary amenorrhea is most commonly caused by

   (A) pregnancy
   (B) ovarian tumors
   (C) congenital abnormalities
   (D) tuberculosis
   (E) lactation

10. The excretion of pregnanediol glucuronide usually

    (A) reaches maximum values during menstruation
    (B) decreases immediately before menstruation
    (C) is uninfluenced by follicle development
    (D) is not related to the menstrual cycle
    (E) varies inversely with progesterone secretion

11. During the climacteric, the urinary excretion of gonadotropin tends to

    (A) increase
    (B) decrease
    (C) vary directly with ovarian function
    (D) remain unaltered
    (E) show unpredictable and great variations

12. In the prevention of cardiovalvular disease in a child who has had rheumatic fever, the most important principle is

    (A) insistence on complete bed rest until the erythrocyte sedimentation rate has returned to normal
    (B) prevention of subsequent attacks of rheumatic fever by drug prophylaxis
    (C) adequate treatment with corticosteroids during acute attacks of rheumatic fever
    (D) adequate prophylactic and restorative dental care to forestall the formation of periodontal abscess or infection
    (E) none of the above

13. A large peripheral arteriovenous fistula should produce a decreased

    (A) pulse rate
    (B) cardiac output
    (C) diastolic blood pressure
    (D) heart size
    (E) venous pressure distal to the fistula

14. A left varicocele which develops after a patient is more than 30 years old and does not collapse when the patient lies supine is indicative of obstruction of the

    (A) pampiniform plexus
    (B) splenic vein
    (C) left renal vein
    (D) vena cava below the renal veins
    (E) left internal iliac vein

15. An appropriate surgical operation is most likely to provide effective relief of ascites when the ascites is secondary to

    (A) cirrhosis of the liver with esophageal varices
    (B) constrictive pericarditis
    (C) tricuspid insufficiency
    (D) thrombosis of the portal vein
    (E) hepatic vein thrombosis (Budd-Chiari syndrome)

16. Following resuscitation from cardiac arrest, a patient is found to have

Arterial pH	7.00
Arterial P_{O_2}	40 mm Hg
Arterial P_{CO_2}	50 mm Hg
Plasma HCO_3^-	8.0 mEq/l
Serum Na^+	145 mEq/l
Serum K^+	6.0 mEq/l

Which of the following statements concerning this patient is most accurate?

    (A) The plasma Cl^- is greater than 110 mEq/l
    (B) The degree of acidosis is determined by the patient's hypercapnia
    (C) The increased plasma K^+ reflects acute renal failure
    (D) The plasma Cl^- is less than 85 mEq/l
    (E) The plasma lactate is greater than 10 mEq/l

17. Hereditary nephropathy may be strongly suspected in the face of recurrent hematuria, a family history of renal disease, and

    (A) deafness
    (B) renal rickets
    (C) azotemia
    (D) bicuspid aortic valve
    (E) horseshoe kidney

18. A 64-year-old diabetic woman enters the hospital with a high fever, back pain, and hematuria. Six months prior to her acute illness her blood urea nitrogen was noted to be 25 mg/100 ml. On admission her BUN is 100 mg/100 ml. Examination of the urine shows numerous gram-negative rods, 1+ protein, 10-25 erythrocytes per high-power field, and numerous hyaline and granular casts. Despite treatment with fluids and antibiotic agents, her fever continues and she develops progressive azotemia. The probable diagnosis is

   (A) acute tubular necrosis
   (B) Kimmelstiel-Wilson syndrome
   (C) renal venous thrombosis
   (D) necrotizing papillitis
   (E) renal cortical necrosis

19. A 65-year-old man, previously well adjusted, began to show a tendency to isolate himself and to be suspicious of others after he had developed tinnitus and progressive loss of hearing. The history suggests

   (A) an early schizophrenic reaction
   (B) organic brain syndrome
   (C) cerebral arteriosclerosis
   (D) psychological reaction to deafness
   (E) none of the above

20. A 36-year-old obese man becomes progressively more elated and excited with increasing capacity for work. He becomes humorous and overactive to the point where it irritates others. He is probably suffering from

   (A) catatonic excitement
   (B) hypomania
   (C) panic reaction
   (D) alcoholic intoxication
   (E) agitated depression

21. Paranoid delusions involve which of the following psychological defense mechanisms?

   (A) Conversion and displacement
   (B) Denial and projection
   (C) Identification with the aggressor
   (D) Isolation and regression
   (E) Repression

22. Which of the following suggests an unfavorable prognosis in schizo-phrenia?

> (A) No obvious precipitating factors
> (B) Abrupt onset
> (C) Intense affect
> (D) Changing symptoms
> (E) Short duration of symptoms

23. If the sensitivity of a screening test for a defined disease is 95 per cent, it may be expected that

> (A) the test will be positive in 95 per cent of individuals with the disease
> (B) the test will be negative in 95 per cent of individuals without the disease
> (C) of the positive individuals, 95 per cent will have the disease
> (D) of the negative individuals, no more than 5 per cent will have the disease
> (E) none of the above is true

24. If the case-fatality rate in a test group receiving a new drug is lower than that in a control group by an amount that is statistically significant at the 5 per cent level, if follows that the

> (A) better results in the test group are attributed to the new drug
> (B) chances are less than one in twenty that the difference is due to sampling variation
> (C) difference could not be due to chance
> (D) chances are more than twenty to one that the difference is due to sampling variation
> (E) drug had no effect on mortality

25. By the application of appropriate statistical techniques to data collected in the course of an experiment, one can usually

> (A) eliminate the influence of chance factors upon the results of the experiment
> (B) estimate the probability that the results obtained could have occurred by chance alone
> (C) reduce the amount of variability present in the data
> (D) control for the effects of sampling errors upon the results of the experiment
> (E) determine whether or not cause-and-effect relationships exist among the variables being studied

26. In an investigation of data on the use of an immunizing agent, the application of a statistical test of significance indicates

    (A) whether the sample size was large enough to provide meaning-ful results
    (B) the extent to which the agent was probably effective in produc-ing any observed differences
    (C) that bias was eliminated
    (D) how often results would differ by as much as the observed difference if chance alone were operating
    (E) the probability that the agent was effective

27. In a child suspected of having acute disseminated histoplasmosis, which of the following tests would be likely to yield the most helpful informa-tion?

    (A) Sheep-cell agglutination titer
    (B) Examination of the bone marrow aspirate
    (C) Skull roentgenogram
    (D) Sedimentation rate
    (E) Widal reaction

28. A 35-year-old farmer sustained a deep puncture wound in his left thigh when he fell on the prongs of a manure fork. You attend him within two hours of the injury, which has produced no serious vascular or neuro-logical problems. After debridement of the wound you should im-mediately administer

    (A) a broad-spectrum antibiotic agent (with the expectation of continuing it)
    (B) 10,000 units of equine tetanus antitoxin
    (C) 16,000 units of equine tetanus antitoxin
    (D) 1 ml of tetanus toxoid and 500 units of human antitetanus globulin
    (E) 2 ml of Clostridium perfringens toxoid

29. Which of the following is LEAST likely to accompany posterior disloca-tion of the hip?

    (A) Aseptic necrosis of the head of the femur
    (B) A chip fracture of the ipsilateral acetabular lip
    (C) Hemarthrosis of the ipsilateral knee
    (D) Damage to the sciatic nerve
    (E) Damage to the femoral nerve

30. Once carcinoma of the lung has been diagnosed, each of the following is usually considered a sign of inoperability EXCEPT

    (A) paralysis of the diaphragm on the ipsilateral side
    (B) Horner's syndrome on the ipsilateral side
    (C) serosanguineous pleural effusion
    (D) marked pulmonary osteoarthropathy
    (E) biopsy of an anterior scalene node that is positive for tumor

31. The probability of postpartum hemorrhage is increased by each of the following EXCEPT

    (A) precipitate labor
    (B) prolonged labor
    (C) multiple pregnancy
    (D) premature rupture of the membranes
    (E) hydramnios

32. Congestive heart failure is associated with each of the following EXCEPT

    (A) decreased renal blood flow
    (B) increased blood volume
    (C) hypernatremia
    (D) increased interstitial fluid volume
    (E) decreased glomerular filtration rate

33. A 48-year-old patient with a history suggestive of an indolent, progressive meningitis of two weeks' duration shows signs of meningeal irritation. Lumbar puncture yields slightly cloudy fluid with 380 leukocytes per cu mm (90 per cent lymphocytes, 10 per cent polymorphonuclear cells); protein 110 mg/100 ml; glucose 10 mg/100 ml. Each of the following etiologic possibilities might be seriously considered in the differential diagnosis EXCEPT

    (A) *Cryptococcus neoformans*
    (B) *Mycobacterium tuberculosis*
    (C) lymphomatous involvement of the meninges
    (D) Coxsackie virus, group B
    (E) carcinomatous involvement of the meninges

34. Each of the following may promote convulsive seizures in susceptible individuals EXCEPT

    (A) acidosis
    (B) hypoglycemia
    (C) excessive water retention
    (D) alkalosis
    (E) withdrawal of phenobarbital

35. Each of the following is associated with intrauterine growth retardation of the fetus EXCEPT

    (A) trisomy 17-18
    (B) rubella
    (C) osteogenesis imperfecta
    (D) cystic fibrosis
    (E) toxoplasmosis

DIRECTIONS: This section of the test consists of several situations, each followed by a series of questions. Study each situation, and select the one best answer to each question following it.

Questions 36–37

A physician is called to an apartment to see a new patient. He finds the markedly jaundiced body of a young woman, whose alleged sister gives the following history. Five days previously the patient, who thought she was pregnant, had gone to see a man who inserted a catheter into the uterus to produce an abortion. Following this, she became very ill. She died shortly after the sister called the physician.

36. The physician should immediately

    (A) call in a consulting obstetrician
    (B) send the body to the nearest hospital for an autopsy
    (C) sign the death certificate, giving the cause of death as "abortion"
    (D) notify the police and await their instructions
    (E) send the body to the nearest mortuary and call the police

37. The most likely underlying cause of death is

    (A) liver failure
    (B) *Clostridium perfringens* septicemia
    (C) acute glomerulonephritis
    (D) *Escherichia coli* septicemia
    (E) *Staphylococcus aureus* septicemia

Questions 38–40

A 28-year-old drug addict is found in his room disoriented and covered with urine and feces. He is withdrawn and refuses to give a history. Physical examination shows a temperature of 40.9 C (105.6 F), a pulse rate of 132/min, a respiration rate of 24/min, and a blood pressure of 120/60 mm Hg. Surface veins of the forearms and upper arms are thrombosed and there are needle marks in both antecubital fossae. The heart, lungs, and abdomen show no abnormalities. He is admitted to the hospital with a presumptive diagnosis of bacterial endocarditis.

38. On the second hospital day, blood cultures taken on admission are reported as positive. The organism most likely to have been grown is

    (A) hemolytic (coagulase-positive) staphylococcus
    (B) *Staphylococcus epidermidis*
    (C) *Candida albicans*
    (D) group A beta-hemolytic streptococcus
    (E) streptococcus, viridans group

39. On the fourth hospital day, a harsh systolic murmur is heard over the center of the precordium, an enlarged pulsatile liver is felt, the neck veins are distended, and an infiltration of the right lower lobe is seen on a roentgenogram of the chest. The most likely explanation is

    (A) pulmonary hypertension secondary to multiple septic pulmonary emboli
    (B) rupture of an aneurysm of the sinus of Valsalva
    (C) purulent pericarditis
    (D) tricuspid valvular incompetence
    (E) mitral valvular incompetence

40. The best way to ascertain the nature of the anatomic lesion is by

    (A) fluoroscopy
    (B) right-heart catheterization with angiography
    (C) right-heart catheterization with determination of pressures and flows
    (D) left-heart catheterization with determination of pressures and flows
    (E) left-heart catheterization with angiography

Questions 41–42

A 32-year-old man was getting gasoline at a roadside service station when a car traveling at a high rate of speed hurtled from the road and crashed into the automobile which the patient had vacated moments earlier. The wreck burst into flame and, anticipating a serious explosion, the patient assisted in pulling the driver from the flaming wreckage. An elderly man who was helping the patient suffered a heart attack and died in the process, and the extricated driver died moments later.

After the patient left the scene of the disaster, he was unable to stop trembling, and he maintained a marked, visible tremor for two months, during which time he had repetitive dreams of fighting his way out of a raging fire which occurred in various settings.

41. The most likely diagnosis is

    (A) hypochondriasis
    (B) anxiety hysteria
    (C) traumatic neurosis
    (D) phobic reaction
    (E) psychophysiological muscle reaction

42. The patient's repetitive dreams of fighting his way out of a fire probably represent

    (A) an attempt to master his anxiety
    (B) his feeling of pleasure in being a hero
    (C) a recollection of childhood incidents of playing with fire
    (D) a wish to punish himself
    (E) psychotic perseveration

Questions 43–45

A newborn infant with an abnormality of the genitalia that appears to be hypospadias is well for a week. Then the infant begins to vomit forcefully and becomes dehydrated. Administration of fluid and electrolytes parenterally in quantities usually sufficient to correct dehydration in a child of this age for at least a day fails to do so. Six hours after administration of the fluids the dehydration recurs, although the vomiting has stopped. A diagnosis of adrenal insufficiency associated with congenital adrenal hyperplasia is made.

43. At the time the dehydration was the greatest, the serum would be most likely to show

   (A) decreased carbon dioxide combining power and hyperchloremia
   (B) increased carbon dioxide combining power and hypochloremia
   (C) decreased carbon dioxide combining power and hypokalemia
   (D) hypochloremia, hyponatremia, hyperkalemia, and azotemia
   (E) no significant change from normal values

44. From the standpoint of diagnosis, the most important abnormality in the urine would be

   (A) marked reduction in specific gravity
   (B) absence or marked decrease of ammonia
   (C) increased excretion of 17-ketosteroids
   (D) marked decrease of chloride
   (E) a strongly acid reaction

45. In addition to parenteral administration of fluids and electrolytes, the preferred treatment would include

   (A) norepinephrine
   (B) vasopressin (Pitressin)
   (C) oral administration of a strongly alkaline electrolyte solution
   (D) ACTH
   (E) desoxycorticosterone acetate, supplemental salt, and cortisone

---

DIRECTIONS: Each group of questions below consists of lettered headings or a diagram or picture with lettered components, followed by a list of numbered words, phrases or statements. For each numbered word, phrase or statement, select the one lettered heading or lettered component most closely associated with it. Each lettered heading or lettered component may be selected once, more than once, or not at all.

Questions 46–49

The graphs below represent the patterns of labor in four different multiparous patients. For each statement that follows, select the pattern of labor most consistent with it, and mark the answer sheet in accordance with the following:

(A) if associated with graph A
(B) if associated with graph B
(C) if associated with graph C
(D) if associated with graph D

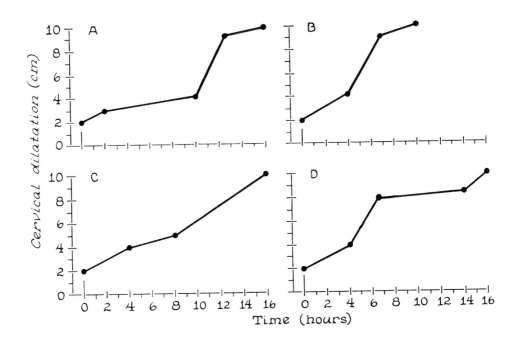

46. Secondary arrest

47. Normal labor

48. Prolonged latent phase

49. Desultory labor

Questions 50–54

Maternal history:

    (A) Oligohydramnios
    (B) Hydramnios
    (C) Toxemia
    (D) Diabetes mellitus
    (E) None of the above

Possible related condition in newborn:

50. Renal agenesis

51. Prematurity

52. Retrolental fibroplasia

53. Macrosomia

54. Duodenal atresia

Questions 55–59

    (A) Aseptic meningitis with a rash
    (B) Herpangina
    (C) Pharyngoconjunctival fever
    (D) Chorioretinitis
    (E) Epidemic pleurodynia

55. Coxsackie virus, group B

56. Toxoplasma

57. Adenovirus

58. ECHO virus

59. Coxsackie virus, group A

Questions 60–62

    (A) Vertical transmission
    (B) Indirect (vector) transmission
    (C) Transmission by a common vehicle through continuous exposure
    (D) Transmission by a common vehicle through a single exposure
    (E) Person-to-person transmission

60. Explosive outbreak

61. Secondary cases

62. Seasonal variation over a limited geographic area

Questions 63–66

       (A) Kanamycin sulfate
       (B) Tetracycline
       (C) Erythromycin
       (D) Chloroquine
       (E) Chloramphenicol

63. May cause hearing loss

64. Outdated material may cause aminoaciduria and renal tubular acidosis

65. May cause hemolytic anemia in genetically susceptible individuals

66. Prolonged therapy may cause proteinuria

Questions 67–70

Listed below are five lettered organs. For each of the numbered diseases that follow, select from the lettered list the organ other than the kidney that is most likely to be involved.

       (A) Lungs
       (B) Acoustic apparatus
       (C) Liver
       (D) Heart
       (E) Esophagus

67. Hereditary nephritis

68. Goodpasture's syndrome

69. Polycystic disease

70. Scleroderma

Questions 71–74

A patient is admitted to the emergency room following blunt trauma to the anterior chest wall. There are multiple fractured ribs on both sides of the sternum. Each of the lettered signs below is an additional finding that may be exhibited by this patient. For each of the numbered diagnoses that follow, select the sign that is most closely associated with it.

    (A) Distended neck veins
    (B) A "sucking" wound
    (C) Paradoxical respiratory motion of the chest wall
    (D) Subcutaneous emphysema
    (E) A difference in blood pressure in the two arms

71. Flail chest

72. Cardiac tamponade

73. Tension pneumothorax

74. Lacerated lung

DIRECTIONS: Each set of lettered headings below is followed by a list of numbered words or phrases. For each numbered word or phrase select

    A if the item is associated with (A) only,
    B if the item is associated with (B) only,
    C if the item is associated with both (A) and (B),
    D if the item is associated with neither (A) nor (B).

Questions 75–76

    (A) Patent ductus arteriosus
    (B) Coarctation of the descending thoracic aorta
    (C) Both
    (D) Neither

75. Widened pulse pressure in the lower extremities

76. Can lead to left ventricular enlargement

Questions 77–81

    (A) Acute post-streptococcal glomerulonephritis
    (B) Acute rheumatic fever
    (C) Both
    (D) Neither

77. Reactivation frequently occurs in association with acquired streptococcal infection

78. Prolonged prophylactic administration of penicillin is recommended

79. Complete recovery without residual organ damage occurs in over 90 per cent of patients under 16 years of age

80. Infections with type 12 beta-hemolytic streptococci are particularly related

81. Electrocardiographic changes are seen

Questions 82–85

      (A) Rheumatic fever
      (B) Rheumatoid arthritis
      (C) Both
      (D) Neither

82. Antistreptolysin-O titer elevated

83. Aortic regurgitation

84. Subcutaneous nodules

85. Therapy with penicillin relieves acute attack

DIRECTIONS: For each of the questions or incomplete statements below, ONE or MORE of the answers or completions given is correct. Select

      A if only 1, 2, and 3 are correct,
      B if only 1 and 3 are correct,
      C if only 2 and 4 are correct,
      D if only 4 is correct,
      E if all are correct.

Directions Summarized				
A	B	C	D	E
1,2,3 only	1,3 only	2,4 only	4 only	All are correct

86. Which of the following may be useful in establishing the diagnosis of hypertension due to unilateral disease of a renal artery?

    (1) Aortography
    (2) Measurement of sodium excretion from each kidney
    (3) Intravenous pyelography
    (4) Measurement of plasma renin activity in blood from each renal vein

87. Intravenous pyelography is dangerous in a patient with

    (1) acute pyelonephritis
    (2) bilateral stag-horn calculi
    (3) an increased blood urea nitrogen concentration
    (4) allergy to iodides

88. Traumatic arteriovenous fistula produces

    (1) a wide pulse pressure
    (2) increased cardiac output
    (3) dilatation and hypertrophy of the left ventricle
    (4) pulmonary hypertension

89. An infant receiving a properly constructed formula of boiled cow's milk, water, and carbohydrate as his sole dietary intake would be prone to develop

    (1) kwashiorkor
    (2) anemia
    (3) beriberi
    (4) scurvy

Directions Summarized				
A	B	C	D	E
1,2,3	1,3	2,4	4	All are
only	only	only	only	correct

90. Situations that tend to enhance the development of a strong ego during childhood include

    (1) exposure to frustrations that are rational and real rather than artificially created

    (2) exposure to frustrations that are, at the time, within the ego capacity of the child

    (3) repeated experiences with desirable substitute gratifications for forbidden and undesirable ones

    (4) minimizing, through explanation and affection, the tendency of the child to interpret reality frustrations as hostile attacks

91. A statistically significant association exists between perinatal traumata and

    (1) behavior disorders of childhood

    (2) hysterical reaction

    (3) epilepsy

    (4) somnambulism

92. In men with severe depressions, symptoms frequently include

    (1) early morning awakening

    (2) nihilistic delusions

    (3) diurnal mood swings

    (4) impotence

93. Compared with a suburban population, the population residing in the center of a large urban area has a significantly higher prevalence of

    (1) depression

    (2) schizophrenia

    (3) anxiety-hysteria

    (4) alcoholism

Directions Summarized				
A	B	C	D	E
1,2,3 only	1,3 only	2,4 only	4 only	All are correct

94. Choriocarcinoma

    (1) in many cases is successfully treated with methotrexate
    (2) will be a sequela of approximately 50 per cent of hydatidiform moles
    (3) can arise following an apparently normal pregnancy
    (4) produces excessive levels of follicle-stimulating hormone (FSH)

95. Palliation in metastatic carcinoma of the breast in a premenopausal woman may be achieved by

    (1) oophorectomy
    (2) hypophysectomy
    (3) adrenalectomy
    (4) administration of 5-fluorouracil

96. Compression of the first sacral root by a herniated lumbosacral disc produces

    (1) numbness of the 5th toe
    (2) absence of the knee jerk
    (3) absence of the Achilles reflex
    (4) urinary retention

97. Oxytocin in humans is

    (1) a normally produced hormone with a polypeptide structure
    (2) rapidly eliminated or made inactive in both pregnant and nonpregnant patients
    (3) most effective at term in augmenting uterine contractions
    (4) released into the circulation as a result of suckling

Directions Summarized				
A	B	C	D	E
1,2,3 only	1,3 only	2,4 only	4 only	All are correct

98. A 13-year-old girl has had irregular, painless periods of uterine bleeding lasting as long as 12 days since the menarche nine months ago. Physical examination, including pelvic examination, shows no abnormalities. In this patient's premenstrual phase

    (1) premenstrual tension is unlikely
    (2) the endometrium is secretory
    (3) the cervical mucus shows a fern pattern
    (4) exfoliated vaginal cells curl and clump

99. Which of the following should not be used or should be used with caution in a patient suspected of having a duodenal ulcer?

    (1) Reserpine
    (2) Phenylbutazone
    (3) Cortisol
    (4) Aspirin

100. Normal immunologic responsiveness is depressed in patients with

    (1) a burn covering 40 per cent of the body surface
    (2) Hodgkin's disease
    (3) chronic uremia
    (4) myasthenia gravis, following thymectomy

Part III—Examples of Questions Presenting Clinical Problems Based on Pictorial Material: Questions 1–18

DIRECTIONS: The questions below are related to accompanying illustrative material. Answer each question by selecting the <u>one</u> best choice.

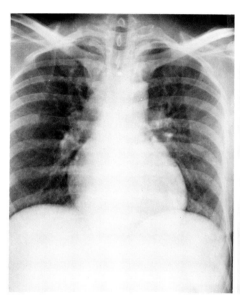
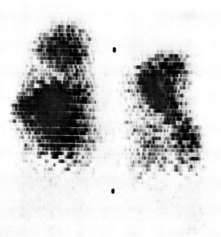

1. The above scan shows

   (A) areas of diminished alveolar ventilation
   (B) areas of diminished pulmonary perfusion
   (C) pulmonary consolidation
   (D) alveolar capillary block
   (E) localized area of overdistention

2. Which of the following is the most likely diagnosis?

   (A) Bullous emphysema
   (B) Pulmonary embolism
   (C) Pulmonary fibrosis
   (D) Pneumonia
   (E) Neoplastic disease

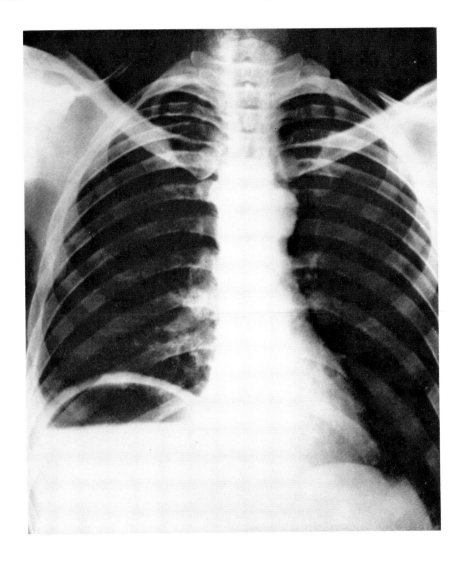

The roentgenogram shown above is that of a 50-year-old man who has had upper abdominal pain, fever and vomiting for three days.

3. This clinical picture is probably due to which of the following?

    (A) Amebiasis
    (B) Suppurative cholangitis
    (C) Ruptured peptic ulcer
    (D) Abdominal situs inversus
    (E) Emphysematous cholecystitis

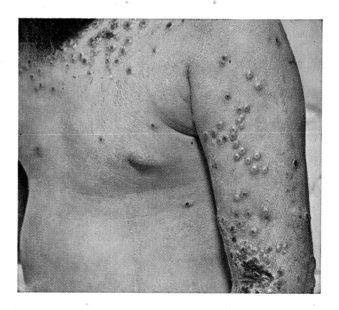

The above photograph is that of a 3-year-old boy who has had eczema for one year. Four days ago he developed vesiculopustular lesions in those areas of the face, neck, and arms where the eczema was most intense. He developed fever and, despite adequate penicillin therapy, new lesions continued to appear. Smears showed questionable intracytoplasmic inclusions but no multinucleated giant cells or intranuclear inclusions.

4. Which of the following statements would be most likely to apply?

   (A) The patient would improve dramatically when treated with erythromycin by mouth
   (B) A sister was vaccinated three weeks previously
   (C) Spherical particles would be found in vesicle fluid by electron microscopy
   (D) An older brother had fever blisters two weeks previously
   (E) Inoculation of HeLa cultures with vesicle fluid would have no visible effect

Questions 5–6

The following chart shows the influence of spironolactone on a 40-year-old man. Examination of the optic fundi showed arteriovenous nicking. Plasma volume was increased. Urinary excretion of 17-hydroxycorticoids (24-hour) was within normal limits.

The dotted horizontal lines on the urine sodium and urine potassium sections indicate the intake of these ions. "S.R." on the chart means secretion rate.

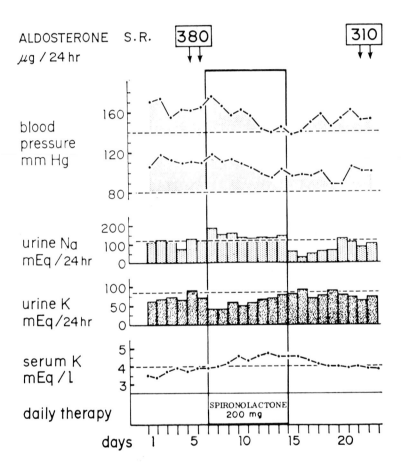

5. Which of the following is the most likely diagnosis?

    (A) Renal vascular hypertension with secondary aldosteronism
    (B) Malignant hypertension with secondary aldosteronism
    (C) Benign essential hypertension
    (D) Primary aldosteronism (Conn's syndrome)
    (E) None of the above

6. The most valuable single diagnostic procedure would be

> (A) renal biopsy
> (B) renal arteriogram
> (C) measurement of plasma renin activity
> (D) split renal function studies
> (E) none of the above

Questions 7–16

DIRECTIONS: Study the four electrocardiograms (A, B, C, D) shown on the following pages. For each numbered word or phrase below, select the answer in accordance with the following:

> (A) if associated with the pattern shown in electrocardiogram A
> (B) if associated with the pattern shown in electrocardiogram B
> (C) if associated with the pattern shown in electrocardiogram C
> (D) if associated with the pattern shown in electrocardiogram D
> (E) if associated with none of the electrocardiographic patterns
>   shown

7. Hyperthyroidism

8. Digitalis is the drug of choice

9. Hypokalemia

10. Hyperkalemia

11. Heart rate varies with respiration

12. History of paroxysmal tachycardia since childhood

13. Commonly found in children

14. Administration of anticoagulants may be of value

15. Digitalis toxicity

16. Paradoxical pulse

Study the four electrocardiograms shown below (A, B, C, D). Then answer Questions 7–16 on page 165.

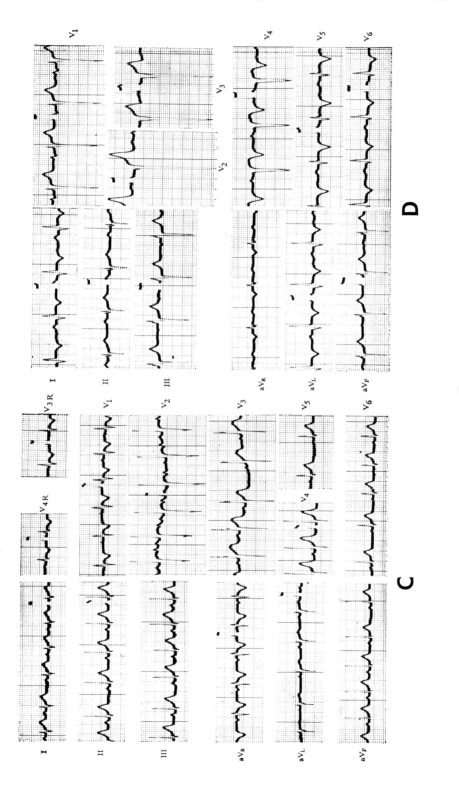

Questions 17–18

DIRECTIONS: The questions related to the pictorial material shown below are examples of the use of such material and item type X. Select each alternative that you think is correct. All, some, or none of the alternatives may be correct.

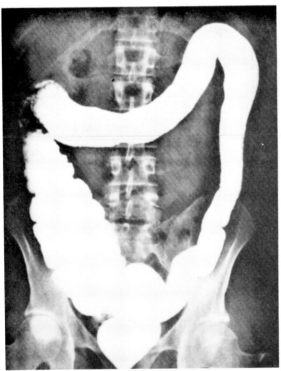 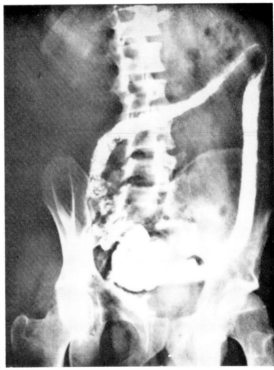

17. Which of the following might be expected in association with the roentgenographic findings shown above?

    (A) Arthritis
    (B) Megaloblastic anemia
    (C) High peaked T waves on electrocardiogram
    (D) Uveitis
    (E) Pulmonary cavitation

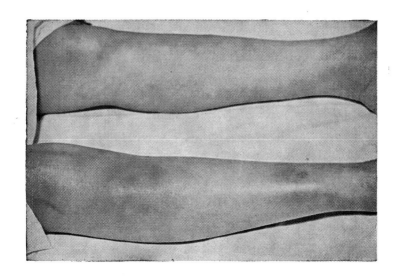

18. The lesions shown above are associated with

    (A) ulcerative colitis
    (B) tuberculosis
    (C) coccidioidomycosis
    (D) sarcoidosis
    (E) primary syphilis

Part III—Patient Management Problems: Questions 1–43

GENERAL INSTRUCTIONS

This test is designed to assess certain aspects of clinical problem solving. You will be given an opportunity to obtain clinical information, to order diagnostic studies and procedures, to make diagnostic hypotheses, to prescribe therapy, and to make other decisions regarding each of a number of patients. Your task is to determine which options you consider appropriate, just as you would be expected to do if you were managing an actual patient.

A series of problems is associated with each patient. For example, the problems associated with Patient A are identified as Problem A-1, Problem A-2, Problem A-3, etc. The problems for each patient should be undertaken in the order in which they are presented.

Initial information is given for each patient. Following this initial information, the first of a series of problems (Problem A-1) for that patient (Patient A) is presented. This problem consists of a numbered list of possible courses of action arranged in random order. You are not told how many courses of action are considered correct; for each problem, your task is to select those diagnostic or therapeutic procedures that you think should be done for this patient at this point in time.

First, read all of the courses of action listed in the problem. Then select a study or procedure that you think should be done. Move across to the identically numbered rectangle to the right of this action and, using the special pen provided, carefully—lightly—rub the area within this rectangle. Within seconds, there will appear printing that designates feedback indicating the result of this action. The end of each feedback is identified by an asterisk (*). Always develop each selected response one at a time until you reach the asterisk (*). The information you receive may lead you to select other procedures within the same problem, or you may decide to make other choices quite independent of results already obtained. After you have completed Problem A-1, and bearing in mind the additional information resulting from your decisions, proceed in a similar manner with Problem A-2, etc.

The response that appears in the rectangle does not necessarily indicate that the choice is correct or incorrect; for correct as well as incorrect choices, the following kinds of responses will appear in the feedback:

(1) When you order a diagnostic study (e.g., blood glucose, electrocardiogram, etc.), or a diagnostic procedure (e.g., liver biopsy, thoracentesis, etc.), specific data may be reported, or the response may indicate that the study or procedure was ordered or done.

(2) When you order a therapeutic measure, the response will usually simply indicate that therapy was given or ordered.

(3) Where the response differs from those listed above, the response given will be self-explanatory (e.g., "Patient refuses operative procedure").

Your score on this section of the examination will be based on the total number of correct decisions that you make. Selecting indicated options and avoiding unnecessary or contraindicated options will improve your score. Any exposure in a rectangle that reveals any portion of the underlying answer will be treated as a selection; be careful not to let your special pen accidentally rest on a rectangle that you do not select.

PATIENT A

There are 5 problems related to Patient A. These 5 problems should be undertaken in sequential order. Choices within each problem, however, may be made in any order.

General Information

A 45-year-old man is admitted to the hospital because of pain in his right hip and pelvis, especially when walking. He had lost 30 pounds in weight in the past year, during which time he did not feel strong or well enough to work. Three months prior to admission, he developed an acute upper respiratory infection and noted an increase in his symptoms with generalized "pain in my bones and stiffness of my joints." At that time, he also noted generalized numbness with tingling and stiffness of his hands; he had difficulty talking because his jaws and lips became stiff, making it difficult to form words.

Twenty years earlier he had had similar symptoms which he described as "pain all over." At that time, he was studied at a hospital for bone and joint disease, where he was told he had "osteoporosis." During the intervening years, he has been relatively well.

Physical Examination

Temperature is 37.0 C (98.6 F); pulse rate is 80 per minute and regular; blood pressure is 120/80 mm Hg. The patient is well developed and appears well nourished. The lungs are clear to percussion and auscultation. The heart is normal in size; there are no murmurs. The abdomen is protuberant but no masses or organs are palpable. There is tenderness in the right groin on palpation but no mass can be felt. There is 2+ edema of the legs but the extremities are otherwise normal. Neurological examination shows no abnormalities. Walking causes severe pain in the right hip and pelvis as well as pain in the feet.

Initial Laboratory Studies

Hemoglobin	10.0 gm/100 ml
Hematocrit	35 per cent
Leukocyte count	6,800/cu mm; neutrophils 60, lymphocytes 34, monocytes 5, eosinophils 1
Erythrocyte count	4,000,000/cu mm
Urine	Specific gravity 1.015, pH 5.5; protein 1+, glucose and acetone negative; microscopic examination: 3-4 WBC, 1-2 RBC per high-power field; no bacteria, casts or crystals
Roentgenogram of the chest	Lung fields clear

Problem A–1

With the understanding that all elements of the history are important, inquiries about which of the following are specifically pertinent with regard to this patient's problem?

1. Appetite   #

2. Consumption of citrus fruits, juice, or foods containing ascorbic acid   #

3. Frequency, volume, consistency, and description of stools   #

4. Transfusions, injections, "needles"   #

5. Exposure to people with cough, fever, or known infectious illness   #

6. Rickets in childhood, intake of vitamin D, exposure to sunlight   #

7. Sore throat, streptococcal infection, evidence or diagnosis of nephritis or kidney disease in childhood   #

If you select this option, turn to page 176 to learn what would appear upon developing this box with the "special pen" in the actual examination.

8. History of hot, red, or swollen joints

#

9. Family history (siblings, parents) of skeletal deformity or "bone" pain

#

Problem A–2

You would now measure

10. serum transaminases

#

11. serum calcium and phosphorus

#

12. serum alkaline phosphatase

#

13. serum sodium, potassium, chloride, and bicarbonate

#

14. blood urea nitrogen

#

15. serum iron and total iron-binding capacity

#

16. serum acid phosphatase

#

17. phosphate clearance

#

18. antistreptolysin-O titer

#

19. bromsulphalein excretion

#

20. serum uric acid

#

#If you select this option, turn to page 176 to learn what would appear upon developing this box with the "special pen" in the actual examination.

Problem A–3

On the basis of your findings up to the present time, which of the following studies would you expect to yield helpful information?

21.   An intravenous pyelogram   #

22.   Roentgenograms of the skeleton   #

23.   A Schilling (radioactive cyanocobalamine excretion) test   #

24.   Determination of fecal fat excretion   #

25.   A glucose tolerance test (oral)   #

26.   A D-xylose tolerance test   #

27.   Cystoscopy   #

28.   Roentgenograms of the small intestine   #

29.   A barium enema   #

Problem A–4

You would now order

30.   a liver biopsy   #

31.   a renal biopsy   #

#If you select this option, turn to pages 176–177 to learn what would appear upon developing this box with the "special pen" in the actual examination.

32.   a bone marrow examination   #

33.   a biopsy of the small intestine   #

34.   an exploratory laparotomy   #

Problem A–5

Therapy would consist of

35.   ferrous sulfate by mouth   #

36.   transfusion with whole blood   #

37.   vitamin D and calcium orally   #

38.   a special diet   #

39.   ammonium chloride   #

40.   a sodium citrate-citric acid mixture orally   #

41.   cyanocobalamine parenterally   #

42.   ascorbic acid orally   #

43.   exploration of the neck for a parathyroid adenoma   #

#If you select this option, turn to page 177 to learn what would appear upon developing this box with the "special pen" in the actual examination.

PATIENT A

Problem A–1

1. Normal *

2. Fresh orange juice daily *

3. Greasy, bulky stools *

4. None *

5. No exposure *

6. No rickets, no exogenous vitamins; normal sun exposure *

7. All negative *

8. None *

9. One sister has arthritis *

Problem A–2

10. SGOT 30 units (N 15–29)
SGOT 40 units (N 9–23) *

11. Calcium 4.6; phosphorus 1.8 mg/100 ml (N 9–11; 3–45) *

12. 58 K.A. units (N 5–13) *

Problem A–2, continued

13. Na$^+$ 142, K$^+$ 4.0, Cl$^-$ 105, HCO$_3^-$ 27 mEq/l (N 137–142, 3.5–5, 98–106, 21–28) *

14. 14 mg/100 ml (N 10–20) *

15. Serum iron 40, TIBC 380 micrograms/100 ml (N 80–130, 288–362) *

16. 1.0 unit (K.A.) (N 1–5) *

17. 23 ml/min (N 5–15) *

18. 125 Todd units (normal) *

19. 5% in 45 minutes (N 5 or less) *

20. 6.0 mg/100 ml (N 2.5–5) *

Problem A–3

21. No abnormalities noted *

22. Generalized demineralization; bilateral pseudofractures of upper femur and scapula *

23. 6% excretion (N > 8%) *

24. 30 gm fat in 72 hours *

Problem A–3, continued

25. | Low flat curve ∗ |

Problem A–5

26. | 1 gm of 25-gm dose excreted in 5 hours (N 5–8) ∗ |

35. | Ordered ∗ |

27. | No abnormalities seen ∗ |

36. | Given ∗ |

28. | Dilated upper small bowel; segmentation and puddling ∗ |

37. | Given; serum calcium and phosphorus rise ∗ |

29. | No abnormalities seen ∗ |

38. | Gluten-free diet given resulting in marked improvement ∗ |

Problem A–4

39. | Given ∗ |

30. | Moderate fatty infiltration ∗ |

40. | Given ∗ |

31. | Normal ∗ |

41. | Ordered ∗ |

32. | Erythroid hyperplasia. Absent iron stores ∗ |

42. | Ordered ∗ |

33. | Flattened epithelial villi; round cell infiltration ∗ |

43. | Done ∗ |

34. | Patient refuses ∗ |

APPENDIX C

■

Answer Keys to Test Questions

Part I—Basic Science Answer Key

1. D	26. A	51. B	76. C
2. C	27. A	52. D	77. A
3. A	28. D	53. E	78. B
4. B	29. E	54. A	79. C
5. D	30. C	55. D	80. E
6. B	31. C	56. A	81. A
7. D	32. E	57. C	82. A
8. C	33. C	58. E	83. B
9. D	34. B	59. D	84. A
10. C	35. A	60. A	85. A
11. C	36. E	61. B	86. A
12. B	37. B	62. A	87. C
13. A	38. A	63. E	88. B
14. B	39. D	64. B	89. B
15. D	40. D	65. A	90. A
16. C	41. A	66. E	91. A
17. B	42. D	67. A	92. A
18. E	43. E	68. B	93. E
19. E	44. C	69. D	94. D
20. E	45. B	70. A	95. E
21. D	46. C	71. E	96. B
22. D	47. D	72. D	97. B
23. A	48. A	73. A	98. E
24. D	49. A	74. B	99. B
25. D	50. D	75. C	100. E

Part II—Clinical Science Answer Key

1. E	26. D	51. C	76. C
2. A	27. B	52. E	77. B
3. D	28. D	53. D	78. B
4. A	29. E	54. B	79. A
5. D	30. D	55. E	80. A
6. D	31. D	56. D	81. C
7. A	32. C	57. C	82. A
8. A	33. D	58. A	83. C
9. C	34. A	59. B	84. C
10. B	35. D	60. D	85. D
11. A	36. D	61. E	86. E
12. B	37. B	62. B	87. D
13. C	38. A	63. A	88. A
14. C	39. D	64. B	89. C
15. B	40. B	65. D	90. E
16. E	41. C	66. A	91. B
17. A	42. A	67. B	92. E
18. D	43. D	68. A	93. C
19. D	44. C	69. C	94. B
20. B	45. E	70. E	95. E
21. B	46. D	71. C	96. B
22. A	47. B	72. A	97. E
23. A	48. A	73. B	98. B
24. B	49. C	74. D	99. E
25. B	50. A	75. A	100. A

Part III—Pictorial Section Answer Key

1. B	10. E
2. B	11. C
3. C	12. B
4. B	13. C
5. D	14. D
6. C	15. E
7. A	16. E
8. A	17. A, D
9. E	18. A, B, C, D

Part III—PMP Answer Key

1. Yes		23. Yes
2. No		24. Yes
3. Yes		25. Yes
4. No		26. Yes
5. No		27. No
6. Yes		28. Yes
7. Yes		29. No
8. Yes		30. No
9. Yes		31. No
10. No		32. Yes
11. Yes		33. Yes
12. Yes		34. No
13. Yes		35. Yes
14. Yes		36. No
15. Yes		37. Yes
16. No		38. Yes
17. Yes		39. No
18. No		40. No
19. No		41. No
20. No		42. No
21. No		43. No
22. Yes		

Index

181

9/2/73-20
6994.